Other books by Violet Weingarten

HALF A MARRIAGE

A WOMAN OF FEELING

A LOVING WIFE

MRS. BENEKER

INTIMATIONS OF MORTALITY

INTIMATIONS OF MORTALITY

Violet Weingarten

ALFRED A. KNOPF NEW YORK 1978

Copyright © 1977 by Victor Weingarten. All rights reserved
under International and Pan-American Copyright Conventions.
Published in the United States by Alfred A. Knopf, Inc., New
York, and simultaneously in Canada by Random House of Canada
Limited, Toronto. Distributed by Random House, Inc., New York.

Most names of people referred to in this book, other than members of the family, have been changed.

Grateful acknowledgment is made to the following for permission
to reprint previously published material:

Mrs. Norma Millay Ellis: from Collected Poems, Harper & Row.
Copyright 1928, 1955 by Edna St. Vincent Millay and Norma
Millay Ellis.

Houghton Mifflin Company and the Sterling Lord Agency: from
"Making a Living" published in The Death Notebooks, Copyright
© 1974 by Anne Sexton, published by Houghton Mifflin Com-
pany; from "Courage" published in The Awful Rowing Toward
God, Copyright © 1975 by Loring Conant, Jr., executor of the
estate of Anne Sexton, published by Houghton Mifflin Company.
Used by permission of Houghton Mifflin Company and the
Sterling Lord Agency.

Little, Brown and Company: from The Ascent of Man by Jacob
Bronowski; from "Dying: An Introduction" by L. E. Sissman,
Copyright © 1967 by L. E. Sissman.

New Directions and J. M. Dent and Company, London: one line
from Dylan Thomas's "Do Not Go Gentle into That Good Night."
Copyright 1952 by Dylan Thomas. By permission of New Directions.

The New Yorker: from "Dying Away" by William Meredith,
published in The New Yorker, October 14, 1974.

The Viking Press, Inc.: from The Lives of a Cell by Lewis Thomas,
Copyright © 1974 by Lewis Thomas.

Library of Congress Cataloging in Publication Data
Weingarten, Violet {date}.
Intimations of mortality.

1. Weingarten, Violet—Diaries. 2. Authors, American—20th
Century—Biography. 3. Cancer—Biography. I. Title.

PS3573.E396Z52   818'.5'403   77-75004

ISBN 0-394-41290-7

Manufactured in the United States of America

First Edition

I first knew Violet Weingarten as a writer—she had written several stories about a "Mrs. Beneker," and I believed that they could be expanded or extended into a novel. While she was doing this, and while the novel was being published, and through the years when her following three novels were being written and published, we became close friends. But this introduction is meant not as a biography of Vi, nor as a eulogy; just as a brief explanation of how the book came to exist, and why so private a statement is being published.

Yet who Vi was helps to explain all this.

First of all, she was *not* Mrs. Beneker—although Mrs. Beneker's curiosity and modesty and intelligence were not unlike Vi's. Mrs. Beneker, apart from anything else, couldn't have written *Mrs. Beneker*—although she could have read it, and thousands of her *did;* with tremendous pleasure. The greatest difference, as I understood it, between the writer and her most famous character was that together with Vi's gentleness and kindness and self-effacing but relentless interest in everything around her, came a very unusual and profound strength—the strength of someone who knew what was really important to her. This strength made her the wife and mother she was, and the friend she was. The same strength equipped her at the age of fifty, despite the self-effacement and the genuine humility, to turn herself into a good and successful novelist.

That strength is what lies beneath this book.

Through two years Vi approached her illness with her emotional and moral strength intact, and with her powers as a writer always at her disposal. She did not know—or acknowledge—how ill she was; and yet, as you will read, she suspected. But fatally ill or not, she was determined to *understand*—and to record. To find the truth and to tell it. To *write* it. As long as she could whenever she could, she kept this journal of her illness. And she knew—she told us so—that it was going to be published; either intact, as it is here, or turned into fiction. In fact, she began to make a novel of this material even as she was experiencing it—a sequel to *Mrs. Beneker* with her heroine, like herself, facing death. The novel never progressed beyond its opening chapters, but the journal was kept assiduously until only a few months before her death. It is the journal of a woman, and a writer, watching herself coping with the increasing possibility of death. And watching herself, almost humorously, turn cancer and death into the objects of her characteristic curiosity.

What will make this journal particularly valuable, I believe, is the remarkable way Vi had, as a writer, in making others identify with her. You could observe this effect in the hundreds of letters she received from casual or not-so-casual readers who had come upon her books in libraries, or summer houses, or in paperback, or through book clubs. These were not ordinary letters of praise to a writer, but letters from people who seemed to feel that in Vi's books their own voices were being sounded. She spoke for them. And it meant a great deal to them that someone did.

That is why I believe this book is important. Among the many fine books about death and dying now being written and published, Vi's seems uniquely to be about ourselves as much as about herself. She could always do that—spin a quiet, delicate bridge of steel between her and you. She does it here, for the last and most meaningful time.

Robert Gottlieb,
Alfred A. Knopf, Inc.

SYLLOGISM

All persons are mortal.

I am a person.

Therefore I am mortal.

(But I don't believe it.)

INTIMATIONS OF
MORTALITY

It begins so simply. There you are walking down the blank corridor toward infinity and suddenly a door looms up ahead of you. How far away it is you don't know, but it's there all right and it's the first time you've seen it. Your chest is caught in a vise, and fire darts down your left arm. You eat a polluted clam. Fall in the bathtub. Walk by a building as a gas main explodes. Or report for a routine checkup feeling like a hypochondriac because obviously you're in perfect health, and the doctor mumbles something about "it" having to come out, no rush, next week will be plenty of time.

Let me tell you about *my* operation. Not much. Just a few notes from the top of the iceberg before it starts melting down. Sickness, like sex, demands a private room, or at the very least, a discreet curtain around the ward bed. It isn't as much fun to write about though. No titillating moments of sublimation. On the contrary. It's scary. Tempting fate. Acknowledging that door. (What's behind it? Harps? Led Zeppelin? Silence?) But it has its uses. Attention should be paid. Look what Kinsey, and Masters and Johnson, did for sex, and the chances are, more of us are mortal than have multiple orgasms. Even now. And unfortunately, as with sex, there's no substitute for the real thing. You really don't know what it's like until you've been bedded.

It's not a matter of jesting at scars without feeling the wound. It's getting an idea of how Mercutio feels after the wound heals. (I know. It didn't. But if there had been an intensive care unit at Verona Memorial, blood plasma, penicillin . . .)

I don't mean how he felt when he was stabbed. That's something else. My guess is it came as a total surprise. Never mind that he dueled with death all the time, and don't tell me about all the little brothers and sisters his mother lost in their cradles, or the

3

friends he lost to the pox or the plague. The fact is it can't happen to you—until it does. And even then, you tend to retort, "Who, me? Uh-uh. Wrong number, bud. All men may be mortal, but I'm a woman, remember. I don't know about you, but I'm okay." Or vice versa. Mercutio was able to toss off that great line about deep wells and wide church doors because he really didn't expect it would serve; it would serve.

I know my first reaction when the doctor frowned, and then explained why, was surprise. And the next was euphoria. You heard me. Euphoria. The shoe I had been listening for—unconsciously—all my life had dropped. The fear that makes me human, my knowledge of my own mortality, the fear I had hidden so resolutely and displayed so obviously (none of us sees his own ostrich rump sticking up there in the air), was suddenly allowed to surface, and I felt an enormous sense of relief. Jumping to an immediate, and premature, conclusion (of course), I was exhilarated at knowing at last what the masked creature looked like. All passion was spent. There was nothing I could do about anything any more. All I had to do was float.

How long did the euphoria last? A minute. Maybe a day or so more. The panic was ephemeral too. Once the actual process of doing something about it begins—the tourniquet, the ambulance, the EKG, the oxygen, the blood tests, the chest X-ray—everything takes place in such a hurried blur, you have no chance to feel anything, much less think about it. You dust off a few tatters—"Ripeness is all," "Nothing to be feared, it is only to be understood," "Yea, though I walk," etc., etc.—every man his own Bartlett; but they fall into shreds before you've been introduced to the night nurse. You're not recollecting in tranquility now, you're tied to the raft, going over the rapids.

Nor is it easy to scatter bon mots among the bedpans, no matter what fantasy you may have improvised for yourself as a patient. Myself, I have always admired the image of Proust dictating changes in his description of the death of Bergotte as he himself lay expiring. I had a little number prepared for my passage to

surgery, and I actually delivered it, I am told, complete with references to Marcel and his faithful Céleste. Unfortunately, I was
already so full of Sodium Pentothal or something that I sounded
like a mildly literate lunatic. Same thing for my post-operative
dissertations. It appears that at my most eloquent I was stoned on
Percodan. By the time they had me down to mild tranquilizers, I
was no longer trying to be an impressive patient, I was just working on being a patient. As long as possible. The hospital (cum
flower arrangements, unreadable books, jolly get-well cards, phone
calls, doting relatives, attentive visitors, et al.) was a safe cocoon.
Outside was Reality. Up Reality.

And then I began to get better. The Great Mother day nurse
began to be cloying and was dispatched. The soiled Hieronymus
Bosch hospital corridor with its amputees in wheelchairs, its post-
ops walking slowly with Foley catheter tubes in their hands, its
food cart parked right after lunch with the night's dinners in its
innards, its uninterested aides gossiping at the central desk with
no ear for the most ingratiating of greetings (never a "Who was
that who just walked by? Oh, that was that nice lady in Room
402, the one who's always smiling!"), the corridor and its fascinating drama turned into an Off-Broadway nightmare, and it was
time to go home.

Which I did.

But not trailing clouds of glory. Oh, no. Intimidated by intimations of mortality.

I had discovered that I was vulnerable. I had had my nose
rubbed in it. Like Job, once "I had heard of thee by the hearing of
the ear, but now my eye sees thee." Heavy stuff. What do you do
with it, aside from trying not to read obituaries? Don't laugh. The
best post-anything advice I can give anyone is to avoid obits like
the plague, for I will tell you, whatever it is you happened to have
had—yellow fever, galloping consumption, smallpox, or failed
brakes—that is what is currently doing everyone in. It does not
make for reassuring breakfast table reading.

As a matter of fact, nothing is reassuring at first, least of all the realization that you did, after all, make it. What is shocking is that you might *not* have. Or that some residue of what hit you remains. A friend of mine who splintered her elbow reaching for a net ball was in a deep depression for months afterward because it was apparent she was no longer going to be able to get to high shelves or slam serves or ignore the damp. Stitches itch, muscles complain, and once a doctor has had a twinge in his chest investigated, he tends to keep his hand on his pulse thereafter.

Your body is suddenly a being apart from you, a traitor, if only because it happened to be sitting too far forward on its seat when the taxi driver made that short stop. And it is a traitor that has to be soft-soaped. Before, the two of you worked together without question. Now you have to get its permission to take it on walks or go to parties or do extra work. You have to give it naps, feed it proteins, promise it that it will get over its hurt feelings, everyone does, it just "takes time," that's what everyone says, ad nauseam, "it takes time."

Well, time is what you have. Minute after minute after minute of it. The here and now. The present. That's all there is, there isn't any more. That's the knowledge we are supposed to have bought with whatever travail we went through. Carpe diem. Live in the present. But what does that mean? Everyone lives in the present. We all belong to Lifers Anonymous, certain only when we reach midnight that we got through one more day without taking that lethal drink. Does knowing it make any difference?

Yes and no.

For a while at least, you find yourself living on two levels. Your husband talks about a trip next year, and you agree, but to yourself, you murmur, "Maybe." You plant perennials in the fall, as usual, but you cannot suppress the thought that you may not see them bloom. It was always true, but now you think it.

You find it hard to make plans. You feel a loss of options. The Greek you were going to study someday, the lover you might take, the house you would have by the sea, the children whose children you looked forward to, the finally successful, definitive book you were going to write—it was all fantasy maybe (or maybe not), and any and all of it might still happen; but everything seems less likely. Life no longer is open-ended. Balloons won't ride at the end of their string forever.

So you realize. But there is a catch. Really to live in the present means abjuring hope, for what does hope imply other than faith in a future? And who that lives is without hope, cliché or no cliché?

Still, as I have said, there is a difference. Or at least there should be. You should have bought a measure of freedom for your pains. You should, finally, be able to sort out what is important to you, and what is not important, and let the latter go by. A sense of mortality can be very freeing.

Unfortunately, sometimes, no matter how you sort, you discover you can't have what you want. Or you don't want it after all, when you see the price you may have to pay for it. Freedom isn't everyone's dish; it can be awfully hard to swallow.

For myself—and it *is* time we get back to Mercutio, isn't it?—I really didn't have to go to the hospital to find out what was important to me. I knew it all along—family, friends, love, work, what else is there? I didn't mourn not seeing the isles of Greece, the stones of Persepolis, the icons of Leningrad, or the tombs across the Nile at Thebes. I've seen them. Anytime anyone asked me to go, I packed. And I didn't regret not spending more time with my children either. Again, anytime they asked me to come, I went. I'm not saying that I am fulfilled, or that I live up to my expectations, or my wants, but I have the same troubles now as before. The fault, dear Brutus, lies not in my scar, but in myself. As always.

What I find myself getting hung up on is minutiae. I have a love-hate relationship with objects. When I got out of the hospital, I was appalled to discover how many things I had. I was glad to see them but I resented their solidity. Silver boxes, ginger jars, topaz inkwells, gold bracelets, turquoise chains, Limoges china—they all had had a life before me, and barring accident (aha!), they would have one after me, no matter how long I might live, and I didn't like the idea at all. It seemed very callous of them.

I'm getting over that first reaction, largely because I don't see the things any more, they're just there, as they've always been. But there are other trivia. If you spend a thousand on surgery, do you boggle at two dollars for a taxi? Do you settle for blue jeans and a shampoo under the shower, having seen the vanity of vanities, or do you ponder French imports and get a super haircut at the hands of the man who does the Duchess of Windsor, my dear? Do you become more compassionate, because you realize what it is to have pain, or at least, to fear it, or do you end up more selfish, because you no longer have to feel guilty for having been immune so long? Do you change your life or try to pick up where you left off?

I haven't the slightest idea. After all, I'm still on the top of that iceberg, although, truthfully, it is melting fast. I suspect that the answer for me is to pick up where I left off and the sooner, the better. If the sight of that door has changed me, it hasn't changed me all that much; even since I started the first paragraph of this meditation, the door has receded a little more. What's more, I live in a world, my world, with people who haven't even glimpsed the door, however close they may be to me. Remember, you have to see it with your own eyes. Borrowing someone else's glasses won't do it. So even if I wanted to change my life, the people I care about aren't going to change theirs. If I want to toss it all away and scuba-dive off the Great Barrier Reef, I'd have to do it on my own, and that I don't want to do. Because I know that the step from the iceberg leads back to an ice floe, and on that floe I'll float, like everyone else, sometimes alone, sometimes alongside, sometimes making small talk, sometimes holding hands, sometimes sad, sometimes happy, always at the whim of the current. Human. Wherever I may be.

Notes from a Left-Hand Desk Drawer

The foregoing came from my left-hand desk drawer—the one into which I toss scraps of paper with notes, jottings, possibilities, and rejected ideas—as opposed to my right-hand desk drawer, in which bits and pieces of the novel I am writing are accumulating (or not accumulating). This has been a year of interruptions —surgery, recovery, death (my mother's, my mother-in-law's), more surgery (my husband Vic's), traumas, tests, more surgery (mine again), recovery, traumas; in short: life. And each time I begin to write the novel again, I am a different person, changed by the interruption, so the novel is not so much an outpouring, which is how it began, but a weaving together of differences, the signposts of a journey during which not only the landscape but the traveler undergoes constant change.

And now, February 4, 1975, I start this, a second journey. (Is it possible for someone to travel two roads at once? Yes, it is.) This one is to be a journal of chemotherapy, and it is fitting that I start it with notes from my left-hand desk drawer because I want it so much to be just that—a left-handed journal, a portion of my life, not the whole, my right hand still committed to the major part of my life, my family and my work.

Still, I have to do some summarizing before I begin. (It's strange. Writing has always been my way of understanding, and coping, but I thought I would write this after the novel. But when Mark—Dr. Markham, the Virgil who with his shining golden bough leads me through the dark wood—suggested I "keep a record," it seemed very right. Two hands at work, juggling, the way I live now, the way I suppose I've always lived, the way everyone lives, but this year I have become very much aware of it.)

The piece which begins this book called "Intimations of

Mortality" was the first thing I was able to write after I began to feel stronger last spring. My agent "loved it." "Besides, Vi," she said, "death is very big now. I'm sure it will be grabbed up." It wasn't. She sent it to Rachel MacKenzie, an editor at the *New Yorker* who has written of her own intimations—open heart surgery—and Rachel MacKenzie sent it back. "Didactic," she said, and I was angry. But rereading it later, I realized she was absolutely right. Not so much that it was didactic as that it was phony. At least, not the whole truth. My mother was alive then, and I didn't want to use the word "cancer." Nonsense, I not only didn't want to use the word, I'm not even sure that I really grasped what had happened to me. I had had cancer, true, but I didn't have it any more. So I generalized. But you can't generalize any of this and make it worth anything. It has to be specific. Not only because I begin to see the same experience is different for everyone, but because it is one thing to have a hysterectomy (benign) or back surgery (like Vic's), and another to have a diagnosis of malignancy. When I say to Vic, "But it seems to me you were active so much faster than I," he says quickly, "It was completely different with me." And it was. Physically harder—after all, it *was* his spine; emotionally (except for not being able to play tennis or put on his socks occasionally), worlds apart. And the slightest hint or comparison between us frightens him.

What that piece was, was whistling in the dark. Pollyanna pretending everything had happened for the best. I got over it. What succeeded that phase was an *idée fixe*—an unending undercurrent—"I think I am well, I am *sure* I am well," and the thought of my *not* being well never leaves my mind. Everything reminds me. I unwrap a toothbrush and think, "Is this my last?" I make a dinner date three weeks hence and wonder, "Will I keep it?" I put on my ragged white country coat and reflect that I really ought to buy a new one, but I know I won't. How can I buy for next winter? I open a drawer and think I ought to tidy it—fast. (Who is going to be rummaging through it when I'm not there?)

A friend arrives with a new friend (his old girl—his wife,

my friend—died over a year ago), and while I welcome her and talk to her and find I like her very much indeed, the inner monologue proceeds: "This is the pattern. I am going to be succeeded by someone younger, prettier, firmer. Does Vic look at them and feel cheated? Does he wish it would be over with me? On the other hand, seeing how it's going to be should make me feel much better. *If* I last, Vic will be pleased, I think that's true; after all, we've been through the other woman bit; if I don't, if he has to go through a period of my being sick, I won't have to feel so guilty about being a burden, because after the pain subsides, and the loss, he will have a chance at a new life again, someone younger, prettier, gayer—so for a year or so of pain, he will buy himself maybe two decades of another good life." Neurotic? I don't know. Have you noticed how quickly widowers, let alone divorced men, remarry, and how happily?

The automatic postscript becomes so burdensome I discuss it with Dr. Markham (not yet Mark to me). As usual, he spends almost an hour with me, and, as usual, when I leave I feel good. Whole. Reassured. This time, again as usual, he says exactly the right thing. He has read my first novel, and he says, "Remember Mrs. Beneker and her quick mind? It's like a computer that ranges over all the possibilities in the space of a second." Something like that anyhow. And it's true. My mind ranges over good possibilities too. Even in that little inner monologue which encompassed so much anger, jealousy, fear, guilt—and then relieved itself of the guilt by the very process.

I have read Stewart Alsop's *Stay of Execution,* and I note that he, too, mentions fear as being always present as "background music." It surprises me too because he seems so strong, so involved, so on top of what is happening to him. My mother dies with a newspaper clipping quoting Shakespeare in her purse—the one about the coward dying a million deaths, the valiant but once. Alsop quotes it too and suggests that maybe it is the intelligent and the imaginative who die a million deaths and the unimaginative who are spared.

—I go to the dentist. Meyer hefts my folder and says, "I've been your dentist for twenty years. Who'll be your dentist fifteen years from now?" What do I feel? A sense of release. I don't have to worry about the future. All my time is found time. I won't be an old lady. En route to Mark's I see the old ladies dragging themselves across the Concourse, and I think the same thought. Joyfully. Still, I have regrets about that, too. I would have been a great old lady—and a pain in the ass, too, I guess, the more of a character I let myself be. Quote La Rochefoucauld: "Age is a woman's hell."

—I take a plane and when it takes off, or lands, I think, "If there is an accident, nobody will realize how lucky it might have been for me," but then I think of the other passengers. Some arranger, God, to arrange sudden disaster for me at the expense of two hundred or so other people. Anyhow, my granddaughters Kim and Polly are usually along. And Vic. What about Bangladesh? Ulster? The stories in the *Times* any day. Let's leave God out of it.

—I wish on a star. "Ten years without cancer." The first fundamental life-or-death wish of my life.

—We leave the East River Drive to exit at Sixty-third Street. I decide that if we make the green light on York Avenue (we have only done so two or three times in the last six years), I shall be all right. Usually we don't. Last night (when this was written), before today's chemotherapy, we did. Q.E.D.

—Kathy, my daughter the doctor (psychotherapist and teacher), tells of an encounter group in which each person wears a metaphorical sweatshirt with inscriptions front and back. Example: Front—*I am a tough independent person;* back—*But I wish someone would take care of me.* My sweatshirt: Front—*All is for the best. I believe;* back—*But I really don't.*

I have a talk with Kathy, one of many. I am torn between a fear of imposing on her, mother leaning too heavily on daughter (as mine did on me), and her obvious desire to have only truth from me. I finally realize it is important to her personally—and *professionally*—for me to be open; it is certainly helpful to me—

and her professionalism gives me an excuse—so this time I tell her of the *idée fixe*. The fear. The thought of suicide. (Not to avoid pain for myself, but to escape the guilt of imposing my dying on her and Vic and Jan—my other daughter—and our friends.) Mostly Vic. Calmly she tells me they discussed it in February (in the months to come I am to learn how much more they knew about me than I did, but at the time, I didn't know anything about it), and that any such thing would be a group decision. The easier thing for them, she says, in the event of—what's the word? I shy away—anyhow, in case, is for me to see it through. Anyway we perceive together that it is an insult to Vic especially, and to the others, to assume they cannot cope with life as it is—it is an insult to me, too. Everyone eventually dies. Why shouldn't I accomplish it as well as the next one? Why not, indeed? I relax. It is all an experience to be experienced; I shall do it as well as the next one.

The fear lifts.

I make friends with the persistent idea. Each time it pops up, I find myself a little amused at its infinite ramifications.

I also collect books and articles on death. I rush to them as if they were sex manuals. I want to find out "how to do it." But then I decide they really don't have much to do with me. I am not dying, even if they did tell you "how to," which they don't, except for Alsop's already famous, "A dying man needs to die, as a sleepy man needs to sleep, and there comes a time when it is wrong as well as useless to resist. . . ."

Better than Millay's "Moriturus" with its "Shrieking to the south, clutching to the north," or Dylan Thomas's "Do not go gentle into that good night." I used to think that was so wonderful, but now I have a picture of a poor old man, wanting to close his eyes, being shaken awake.

So I file away the lists of books for future use, including a poem called "Dying Away" by William Meredith, dedicated to Freud: "He told us/it is impossible to imagine our own deaths/he told us, this may be the secret of heroism." But the same poem tells how Freud asked his friend Schur for two centigrams of morphine, and Freud himself said in 1922, when he was sixty-six: "On 13 March of this year I suddenly entered real old age. Since then the thought of death has never left me." What made him enter real old age? Did he have his cancer then? I remember his saying he would have killed himself sooner except for his wife and his daughter Anna. It just strikes me. That *idée fixe* again. Et tu.

Also for future reference I file away an article on death by chance, death by choice. I buy a book called *Denial of Death* by Becker, which won the Pulitzer Prize, and tear up the gaudy dust jacket so Vic doesn't notice the title of the book so quickly, but although Becker was dying when he wrote it, I don't find it has what I want at all. Sort of early Masters and Johnson treatise. No how-to-do at all.

(Mark, at one of our visits—they're always the same, so I don't go into them: examination, reassurance, some philosophy, out feeling fine—anyhow, at one of them, I ask whether eating well, thinking right, etc., can affect how long we live. He mentions the possibility that how long any of us may live is written in our particular genetic code. The thought enchants me. Predestination. Everyman's fate bound about his neck. Every religious and philosophical concept translated into biological terms. Also, if it's fore-ordained, *one is no longer responsible.* Cancer is the mark of Cain on Abel's head. It draws a circle around you. Death's head at the feast. *Even if you don't hate it any more. As I don't.* Still, if it's been predicted . . .)

A lovely book—*The Lives of a Cell.* Comforting. As Jeremy Bernstein writes in a review of another book by a geneticist, one feels better reading it—"in possession of an enlarged perspective on who one is and on one's place in the natural order and scheme of things."

At the end of my post-Thanksgiving visit, inspired by my correct diagnosis as psychosomatic of the stomach aches occasioned by my father's "weekend" visit (which turned out to be three weeks), Mark says, "If I were to say how I would like Violet Weingarten to be, this is how I would find all the tests."

I have not been scared in a real sense since Vic's operation last August. Taking care of him and our interrelationship (bad at first, wonderful at the end) had ended my patient-hood. But when Mark expresses his pleasure, I get a chill, and I see the evil eye staring gleefully from the wall over his shoulder.

Nevertheless, he says—and the eye winks—he is going to order some tests that he intended to have done in January anyway. We are scheduled to go to Hawaii January 10. I do not buy so much as a bathing suit or a new toothbrush. I *know* we are not going.

And so the tests go on and on. The nuclear ones this time are not frightening, because the doctor talks to me and the room is not darkened. All clear. The upper GI. Clear, too, in the testing room. Then Dr. Ben from the nuclear medicine department catches me in the hall and says, "I'll have to level with you. There's a shadow on one of the X-rays."

My reaction. Shock. For a minute or so. Then calm. I make a pact with myself. If I can manage not to tell anyone, not even Vic, until after Christmas and New Year's, it will turn out to be nothing. I last two days with Vic. Then I tell him. He pales. I ask him not to tell Jan, or Kathy, whom we are going to visit in Boston the next day. (Later, I found out he did tell them.) Mark, as usual, is calm, honest, reassuring. But when I tell him I am not afraid, he exclaims, "Why not, for God's sake? I'm even afraid to check in for a hernia operation." "Well," I say, "I have a good surgeon, and a good you. . . ."

Denial? Sure. But I really have no panic and no need for Valium. In part because the thing that I have been waiting for has come upon me. I was always waiting (after all, I never expected to go to Hawaii). Now it has been spelled out, it doesn't seem so bad. At least, it seems manageable. And there is the magic. I feel I'll get over this one, too. I always need *two* near-misses—in everything. Nothing ever comes easy for me, but it does come eventually. I make another deal, inasmuch as I have broken the one about not telling. If I get over this, I will go and sin no more—

that is, I will not live each day in fear, but treasure it. The glass is half full, not half empty.

Then, one day, it hits me that again I am play-acting—a little. I am indeed trapped. There are no miracles, as I thought the first time. (I walk in off the street, after all, symptom-free, to a strange gynecologist, and he pokes and says, yes, this has to come out; suppose I hadn't gone, isn't that a sign of something benevolent watching over me?) There is nothing to be pleased about. Just ten months, and I am not symptom-free, I have a shadow. ("Yea, though I walk through the valley of the shadow of death . . ." Aha. I find another miracle. I am not going through the valley of death, it is only the "shadow" of death. Footnote: I go to see my surgeon for a checkup after the surgery and see slung on the wall behind him, a jape on the "valley of the shadow" verse which ends, "for I am the biggest son of a bitch in the valley!" Hah.) So it has to be played out. The question is, how well is it played? Same question with everything. Darcus is cleaning outside my room, and she is singing a song about a mountain. Yes, indeed, Lord, I don't ask you to move the mountain, just give me the strength to climb it.

I think of my mother, dying at eighty-three (how I failed her at the end, and resented my having to, and wanting to, fail her because I couldn't come down, I wouldn't come down, using my surgery as an excuse), and telling Kathy, "No matter how much time you have, it isn't enough!" I think of this year. A madness! Cancer, threat of bankruptcy, sickness, death, Vic's back, and more, much more, and yet—and yet, despite it all—I *enjoy* more than I ever did, Vic and I get along better than we ever did; it is in many ways the happiest year of my life. If a year like this is worth it, then life is worth living. It passes understanding.

Christmas is absolutely lovely, so is our vacation in Sarasota with Kim and Polly. I am not play-acting; it is so. No Valium, no night sweats, no overwhelming fear. It is probably limited. Mark says so. Then it is controllable, unlike a mass. I won't think of the bad parts. I have trouble with the notion of God. If you give up the notion of a malevolent one—the evil eye, say—do you have to give up the idea of a good one? I had lunch at some point with Edna O'Brien, who talks of her fear of death. I am not afraid of death, I say, and I'm not; it's the dying I mind, let me die in my sleep like my mother and my grandmother, of a quick heart attack, and that would be all right with me—but, oh, evil eye, and all ye gods that haunt this place, don't listen to me, please, because I'll get my wish and die of a heart attack as I am wasting away with cancer, I know you, I mean die of *nothing else,* just to end, as in the story I wrote about my grandmother, "De Senectute" (no place for it here, I'll make it a footnote somewhere). But Edna says, "Jesus, Mary, it's the afterwards that haunts me, the hellfire and damnation," and I say, "How can you believe in a God like that, one that punishes his children for ordinary human behavior? Would you punish your children that way?" She appears shocked. "But I never think of myself as a grownup, as a mother with God, only as my father and my mother's bad girl. Of course I wouldn't hurt Sacha . . ." Still Bangladesh. The evil eye. Cancer. The Holocaust. Job. He was really dreadful to Job. Without God, on the other hand, without magic, you're on your own. So? I read some of Huxley's biography. "Let go, let go," he says to Maria, dying of—what else?—cancer. Oh, yes, but hold on, hold on, too —the trick is to know when to hold on, and when to let go. Ripeness is all.

So the Monday after New Year's I go to the hospital and have my angiogram. (Last year I wished for it to be the "year of me"—alas, how I got my wish. This year I forgot to wish for anything. Good.) I am a patient, the doctor says—"best in a thousand I've had." "Go on," I say, "I'll bet you say that to all your patients." But the pictures are good—and all clear. And the process, not dreadful. Does trust have anything to do with it? It was like having a surge of hot lava course through me each time. But the doctor was careful to say how long it would be every time, and I would try to lie as quietly as possible, and I would whisper, "Into thy hands I commend my spirit," and count, and it would be over.

Into whose hands? The doctor's? Mark's? My mother's? (After all the newly acknowledged angers and resentments, I suddenly have a sense of her ministration and understanding surrounding me. I suppose I've internalized her again. Loving mother. Loving God. Why not?)

And then I have the surgery, and the first thing I see is Jan, smiling (always Jan, kooky, bottled-up Jan, always turning out to be the strong one, and the one to tell me—she did last time too when I finally got around to asking what they had found). "They didn't take anything out, Mommie, it's all right," and even hurting and half awake, I realize how I would have hated a resection. I never let myself think about it, not really, and now the thought of it shatters me. This time around I am not stoned on Percodan and Valium (different nurse? different circumstances?) and, three days on, I wake up crying. Depressed as I have not been consciously since last February. Not only because of an altercation between Vic and me (which is shortly, and satisfactorily, cleared up—I am very, very sensitive these days, or, as I've said before, maybe freer to express what I feel), but because I think I have been slit open unnecessarily. I am a victim of super-medicine. I could have been in Hawaii, and no trouble to anyone, if I, and everyone else, had kept his mouth shut. The surgical resident comes in. It is seven a.m. "Do you want to be a surgical resident," I ask him, "or do you want to hear about my feelings? I'm very depressed. Shall I give in to it, or should I turn it off?" He looks at me like a surgical resident. Like Gleidman, my surgeon and his mentor. Straight in the eye. "You're depressed," he says, "because you don't know what's going on with you. The professors haven't been clear. I heard them." So he tells me. "Thank you," I say. "Don't mention it," he says, "I'm a nobody so I don't have to futz around." Vic calls. It is eight a.m. I ask him if I can tell him why I am depressed, he says, "Please do," and he listens, and he tells me that they—he, Kathy, Jan, etc.—have known all along that the first ovarian tumor wasn't primary, and that is why Mark has been so super-careful and why they had to go in and look. And then Mark comes in and explains some more. "You're a very unique woman," he says, and as far as I can make out, they have found that my own immunity response encapsulated the cancer cells which were the "shadow" on my colon; like a guinea pig in a laboratory, I rejected the "implant," there is nothing in the literature about it, and I don't know what boggles me more, the fact itself, or that Vic kept it to himself for eleven months, while I was able to manage my secret for no more than two days. (Again, as I write, I see that it is the "rejection" I seized on, not the presence of malignant cells.)

And so I leave the hospital the second time in less than a year, after never having been sick at all before. A "sick" wife for the first time, although I feel much stronger than I did leaving the last time, because for the first time, encapsulated or not, I know there is something "there." Or, at least, *at times,* so I perceive it. And I suspect I am probably going to have the chemotherapy I escaped the last time. I feel shy about coming home this time. I am *not* going to be an invalid. I am *not* going to give in to weakness. For this time it is not "temporary," but permanent. I have, the surgeon tells me by way of farewell, a "chronic disease, like emphysema, no problem, if it flares up again, we'll take it out." Thanks a million.

Still, for the first few days at home, I am euphoric. Entranced, as the last time, at my great good luck. It takes me nearly a week —and another talk with Kathy, down from Cambridge for a visit —to realize it would have been better to have no cancer than just a little, no matter how encapsulated it may be. (Is *that* my situation? I slip in and out of understanding like a man first riding a wave and then diving under it.) Certainly the question remains— is the glass half full or half empty? I guess both, depending on my mood. But always the same glass.

Next Monday I will go to see Mark and he will let me know the decision about chemotherapy. I know what it will be, of course. To do it.

End of introduction to the left-hand desk drawer journal. I have indeed become the long-winded lady. It's the switch from third to first person. I got drunk on it.

Series 1

I see Mark and at first I feel a strain, sitting on the other side of his desk. Our relationship has changed. (One of my first reactions after the bad GI report was that I had let Mark down. He would be disappointed that I hadn't just sailed along.) I feel like a patient now, not like a *possible* (if he should find something in one of his painstaking examinations) patient. There is a new, heavy reality in the office.

I ask him to tell me again what it is that the surgery found, and he asks me instead to tell him what I think my situation is. I do, and he says that is exactly right. Then he draws a careful diagram, shows me where the surgeon sliced for his biopsies, and says, again, "You're a unique woman."

"From such uniqueness," I point out, "you could die," and he nods, but he adds that it is better to be unique in my particular way than in any number of others he could name. True enough. In passing, I tell him what my psychiatrist friend Michael said when I told him what I had discovered, post-surgery (something, it turns out, he had known all along): "Are you angry at me for not telling you?" Michael thought that I should have been told.

Well, says Mark, what do I think? Am I angry at *him* for not telling me the entire truth? Without waiting for me to answer, he goes on to explain how difficult it is to know what to do in situations like mine, and, I suppose, in most situations.

"But you did exactly the right thing," I tell him, and I still think it's so. *Certain* uncertainty would have served me not at all, especially since I was so uncertain anyhow. Anyone but a fool would be. As my long-winded introduction shows, I worried anyhow. No matter how much I said "I had cancer, but now I don't have it any more," I knew the situation could change at any moment. Why else was I going up to Van Cortlandt Avenue East every month? For the same reason, I don't ask too many questions. At least I don't think I do. Not specific ones. Coping ones, yes, but that's different. I don't ask the reason for all the blood tests, or what they are, although I suspect the C in CBC stands for the obvious, and I try not to ask about possibilities. Essentially there is only one question I want answered, and Mark can't answer that one. Great are the uses of ambiguity. Maybe that is a mark of maturity —being grateful for uncertainty.

Besides, this almost-year of grace was very important in my private timetable. Maybe I had my first symptom—the small lump in my shoulder, or another somewhere else I don't know about— two or three years ago, but with my personal life the way it was, it would have been pure disaster to have had it diagnosed. Then a year later I stained—and maybe it could have been, should have been, diagnosed then—but then too it would have been a disaster. (I would have felt Vic was tied to me not by choice but by my illness. I don't think I could have stayed, or if I had, and I probably would have, I would have despised myself for doing so.) And now we had the almost-year "when I didn't know the whole facts," but no one else did for sure either, and so I didn't have shots and pills, and except for my private monologue, I could appear and feel whole, and we could strengthen what we had been able to start to rebuild. Yes, I am very grateful that I was not told the entire story. (Personal, this last? Of course. But as I said, unless it is specific, it is meaningless.)

And now Mark becomes very businesslike. Treatment starts next Monday, he says. Abruptly, as if he is afraid I am going to protest. I should not have any untoward reactions. Yes, I can go away when the series is over.

"Well," I say, "it would be lovely if I could just walk away and forget about the whole thing, but I can't, and in your place, I would make just that decision." Actually I would be uneasy if he had decided against chemotherapy. I ask him just one question. Will what they have decided to give me interfere with what my own body is doing to reject the cells? The medication is being prescribed with exactly that consideration in mind, says Mark.

I embrace him when I leave. We are back where we were before the second surgery.

I go home, call Vic, tell him, he says, "We'll roll with it." I tell Jan. My sister-in-law Edith. A few friends. I am torn between feeling that this is a time for secrecy—why underline the mark of Cain/Abel?—and feeling that if it's not such a big deal, why make a mystery? Besides, life is life.

I lie down and out of nowhere I have a kind of epiphany. I think of how strange it was that I went to the strange gynecologist in the first place, of how Mark ordered the tests months before he would have ordinarily (maybe it kept us from Hawaii, but it also may have introduced the pills and the fluids to kill the cell that popped up in January, say—oh, Mrs. Candide!). I think of how Kathy called Vic the day I had the GI test to tell him she was suddenly worried about me (two days before I told him), and of how he was annoyed at her and told her of course it had come out all right (how is it she had not worried about any of the other tests she knew I had been having?). I think of how I seem to have healed myself, or so the newly benign mother (the Christian Scientist who would have been praying for me, *is* praying for me?) would have phrased it, and my eyes fill with tears of joy, and I call my Christian Scientist sister in California and tell her of the sense I have of being cared for and nurtured, and that even the pills and shots that will be given me will be given with love, and she says, "Of course," and that the acacias, our mother's favorite tree, are all in bloom in Los Altos, and that, of course, her spirit is all around us.

(Odd footnote to the above: Once, while talking to my sister months after our mother's death, she exclaimed, "My God, what's this?" paused, and then said into the phone that Woody, her husband, had just noticed a piece of paper fluttering down— from where?—under their bed, retrieved it and found it to be written on by our mother. Jean read it to me and then sent it on to me. I have just read it again. *Love has no morbid thoughts,* it says, in her quavery old-lady handwriting, *love's presence antidotes every sense of poison.* Her underlining; but chemotherapy equals *poison,* my thought at the moment. There is more. I am feeling very tired, wondering how I will cope in the weeks to come. *Signs of mental equilibrium* says the slip of paper, *are self-poise, reliance that faces things others flee from, strength sufficient for each day's demand when each day's work alone is considered . . . what God cannot do, man need not attempt.* Mary Baker Eddy, I guess, but even so . . .)

Two days pass after Mark said I am going to have chemo-therapy. I begin to wake up with sweats and nightmares. (The first of the starting-all-over-again dreams takes place now. I am nineteen or twenty, I am somewhere in the Catskills, I have to start all over, dating, looking for a man, I have especially to find the young medical student I was in love with years ago, I have to make my life. "But I have cancer," I say, waking up, "I don't have to do it any more, I've done it." I am relieved, and so tired I liter-ally cannot open my eyes for a while. Vic is taking Valium at night, I notice. "It's not me, is it?" I ask. "It's that real estate thing?" "Of course," he says. My widower friend, the psychiatrist, calls to tell me he is going skiing with the young woman I like so much (skiing? set-in-his-ways Michael?), and he wants to know how things are with me. I tell him I am going to have chemo-therapy. "How do you feel about it?" I figure I ought to tell him the truth. As of this moment, uneasy. "I don't blame you," he says. (I explain to myself that I make him uncomfortable—he is going skiing, while I am trapped.) My doctor friend Phyllis calls. I tell her. "Ugh," she says. "It can be very icky." (Everyone has a different reaction to the shots, I tell myself; she can't know any more than I do. Anyhow she's in public health.) My friend Jane says not to worry, her cousin feels lousy for only a couple of hours in the car coming back. My friend Helen reminds me of a woman we know of in the country who has had chemotherapy for ten or fifteen years, so far as we know. She takes her little bottle with her where she goes, and she goes a lot—China, Russia, Africa. She is sick for a day, and that's that. *She* manages.

By coincidence, someone I have not spoken to in years calls. She is a nurse, married to a Haitian doctor, and she tells me one of their friends from Haiti has been living with them for months while he has been treated by the great Dr. Markham. As it happens I have been in several offices where this patient's name has come up—in the hallway of nuclear medicine, Mark's office, X-ray —and I surmise he is *really* ill (as opposed to me who am *not really ill*). I cannot resist telling her I am to be treated too, although I know I shouldn't, and she is both reassuring and frightening. She will come right down to see me and tell me all about it. "I know so much about it," she says, "no matter how bad it is at first, they can adjust it." (But we're not the same; our situations are totally different. I know. I saw his scan. How did that happen? I was shown what a typical *bad* scan looked like. Sorry.)

The February 1975 *Atlantic* arrives, and it has an article written by a man who has had malignant melanoma. Not as philosophical as my rejected pages, and much more specific, but the same failure of nerve. The thread is a surgeon's remark that if the melanoma is in the axillary node, the patient will be in the "Big League." But fortunately, there turns out to be no melanoma in the axillary node, and the writer says joyously, "But I knew it already. I wasn't going to be in the Big Leagues. Not this season." Pure whistling in the dark. I wonder how long it took him to start waking up, wondering.

The melanoma story is followed by one headed "Prognosis," written by a doctor named Martin E. Plaut. Says he sternly: "The man whose melanoma was removed should stop jogging, hitch up his pants, and realize that no certain cure exists for any form of cancer affecting mankind." Also: "Many antitumor drugs kill cancer cells effectively, but cause moderate to dangerous depression of normal white blood cells as well as gastrointestinal upsets and a host of other side effects, ranging from hair loss to heart muscle damage. Cancer chemotherapy is often as difficult to practice as it is for the cancer patient to tolerate."

Two new theories:

1. A pox on medical articles. They don't help the non-sufferers and they sure as hell don't help the sufferers.

2. A pox on use of the word "cancer" as a metaphor, as in: Watergate, a "cancer" on the White House; it (anything) spread its tentacles "like a cancer"; etc., etc.; or as a symbol of failure, as in: man has yet to find a cure for, etc., etc.

On Friday morning, the Friday before the Monday treatment is to begin, I wake up, start to brush my teeth, and throw up. My hairbrush seems unusually full of hair. A sister-in-law died of Hodgkin's disease thirteen years ago and itched all the time. I note that my back is unusually red where I rubbed my towel.

Vic tells me he will go with me on Monday and has rented a car for the occasion (ours is in the country). "I want to talk to Markham anyway," he says. "A woman I was talking to tells me there is an article in the upcoming *Lancet* that says hair loss is reduced if a tourniquet is put around the head at time of injection."

If hair falls out because of interference with hair cells, what good would a tourniquet do?

I think of my friend Frances. She has a plate in her head which slipped some years ago, and her surgeon suggested she tie a cloth tightly around her head each night to push it back. It worked. She had had a mastectomy and a hysterectomy (benign), and in the years since has been more active, resourceful, kinder, and, when life allows her to be, more serene than ever before. She also is beautiful. What would she say if I told her about chemotherapy? Nothing.

Monday comes.

. .

February 3. I have a slight cold, laryngitis, a cough, the first ailment I have had since my surgery last February. Psychosomatic?

Mark asks how I am. I tell him, "I feel nauseated, and I have lost all my hair." Maybe he doesn't hear me. Anyway he doesn't smile. He asks me if I have a general practitioner. Peculiar. I point out that two doctors—one in the country, one in the city, both friends of his and mine—were to have been kept informed about me, but I haven't needed them for anything, and it turns out they haven't called to check on me (pride? lack of interest?), so they haven't been told anything.

"Is there any reason you want me to have a doctor on call now?" I ask tentatively.

"No," says Mark, "but I don't know what is going to happen to you in the next twenty years." He is emptying out a bottle of pills and preparing an injection as he says the last.

I grin. "Did you plan to say that?" I ask him.

He looks genuinely puzzled. "No. I don't know what you mean."

Medicine is an art. I've always thought so. Only an artist would mention the "next twenty years," flipping out the first of my chemotherapy pills. (He has his own *idée fixe,* I suspect that too, but that's one reason why he's so tuned in. Plato's ideal doctor, remember? Feeling in his own flesh . . .)

So I drink the pills and water down, but first I make a toast that is not a usual one with me—*L'Chaim,* To life—and I mean it. Then I have some blood taken out, and something injected in.

Vic comes into the office, we sit for a half hour or so, I wait for something to happen, but nothing does.

I am to have three pills daily before breakfast for the next five days; five weeks hence, repeat. Two injections next Monday. Same the following Monday.

Any special diet?

No.

Vitamins?

Yes. Theragran, two a day. Later on, one a day. "You have had a lot of traumas, the tests, the surgery, the chemotherapy. You can take Valium too. Every four hours." I don't need the Valium. But it is balm to know that I am entitled to feel shaky.

What shall I do about nausea?

Nothing. Some people feel more comfortable with Compazine around, but he really doesn't think I will have any. "I'm not trying to psych you," says Mark, "I really think so."

I know he does, and I believe him.

"May I come up for my shots alone? *Can* I?"

"Absolutely. And go anywhere you like afterwards. Go shopping at Gimbels, if you like."

Gimbels? Who shops at Gimbels? Bendel's, maybe. Bonwit's. I'll bet his mother shopped at Gimbels.

Eventually I arrive home. I am not sick to my stomach, I am starved. So I eat. We have arranged for me to pick up a cooked chicken for dinner because obviously I will not be able to prepare food. I call Vic's office and leave word that I am not cooking because I want to go out. So that night we go to a neighborhood pub and have calves' liver, both of us (verboten for Vic because of his low-cholesterol diet), and steins of beer.

In between my coming home and dinner I have written maybe sixteen pages of this.

The only symptoms I have had so far were a sensation of flushing when I got home and a sinus headache, obviously from my cold.

Day 2. I take my three pre-breakfast pills. I have a sense of foreboding before I do and suddenly think of something my sister-in-law Edith said: "You deserve therapy." Right on. It's not a punishment to be taking these little white pills, it's a privilege.

But I am suddenly very tired. Almost since I got out of the hospital I have been going out to dinner, taking walks, marketing, writing. I look at the calendar. It isn't four weeks since I was slit open. It is time to stop proving things. I go back to bed and at ten a.m. I actually fall asleep. In the afternoon I have my hair done (I had asked Mark if I could dye my hair, and he said yes). At night I get dressed up, really dressed up, and we go to a black-tie foundation dinner at the St. Regis. I see many people I haven't seen for years. No one sees any difference in me, or says so anyway, only that my hair looks great.

Is my hair going to fall out?

Well, I have a lot of it.

Day 3. I took my pills and my vitamins. And having gotten so far up to date on my left-hand desk drawer, I now turn with not a little fear to my right-hand desk drawer. It's not only that I'm physically tired of typing, it's that I wonder who is going to be tackling that novel now. The week of anticipating chemotherapy was still another hiatus.

Day 4. Saw Albee's *Seascape* last night. Middle-aged couple on the beach. He says they've "had" a good life. She wants to live "now." Go from beach to beach. Explore. "What do we have to be afraid of, except cancer or a heart attack?" (I can feel the chill in the aging audience. Heart patients mostly, I suspect.) Again, a sense of no options. Still it takes two giant lizards to shake them, healthy, out of their complacency. Where could I go, well or not, unless I went alone? Vic has his work to do. And even alone, where? A beach isn't what I have in mind; it's Rome, twenty years ago.

I take my pills. I am supposed to make an appointment to see the gynecologist. Routine checkup. But I am in no hurry to do so. What for? Whatever can be done is being done. I feel more secure!

(Footnote: Looking back over what I've written, I see I've left out all the recovery pains of last spring and summer. I forgot how my left leg hurt so sometimes I could hardly walk, forgot that it is only recently that I can fasten my bras or put on my coat without favoring my right arm. It's as though it hadn't been.)

I do call the surgeon to make an appointment. Month-after checkup. Next to Mark, Yang and Yin. Or mirror-image. Something. Even over the phone, Gleidman's self-confidence grabs. "May I drive?" "If you could drive before, you can drive now." Hah! I explain I am having chemotherapy, ask if it would be convenient for me to come to the hospital afterward. "Oh," says he, "so they did decide to give it to you. On again, off again Harry." I feel good. If there was still a question . . . (Little goblin interjects: "Maybe because they didn't think it would matter." Up yours, little goblin, I know that's not so.)

Day 5. The last of the pills. Not to think about (I hope) for four more weeks.

Nothing to report. That would be the best part of this journal, wouldn't it? Nothing to report.

Week 2. Monday. Two injections.

Mark, masked, not feeling well, but also noncommunicative. (Typing this—how could he communicate wearing a mask?) It is as if, shots being given, we're out of the realm of choices. No reason to examine me (of course, it's only weeks since I've left the hospital); all that can be done is being done.

My friend Ruth's curious statement yesterday: "Doesn't it give you a funny feeling to think the doctors are experimenting with you?"

Gleidman's comment on above: "They'd be experimenting if they *didn't* give you chemotherapy."

One man's meat.

A woman in Mark's office is making an appointment for a checkup in February of 1976! For a mammogram too, so it must be post-cancer. Marvelous.

I arrive back at the apartment at three p.m. I waited in twenty-degree, or less, cold for the bus, which was an hour late.

I am hungry, as I was last week, and about an hour or so later, I feel the flush.

Only untoward symptom during the week, I note, was feeling of fullness, gas, extension of abdomen after eating. Gleidman, seen after Mark, says this is lack of muscle tone. I should do sit-ups, even though they hurt my pinched nerve. I think maybe it's the super-dose of vitamins. Unimportant either way.

Day 2. I am full of anger this morning.

I am angry because I spent so much time waiting in the cold for the downtown bus. Why did I do it? Is the ten dollars I spend on a taxi going to matter when I'm gone? Don't we—okay, Vic—spend hundreds on plane trips for the kids, presents, etc.? I'm para-noid. I didn't know the bus was going to be an hour late, it wasn't all that cold, and besides the entire Concourse was lined with old people, also waiting in the cold, and the Montefiore corner is sunny.

Why am I angry? Maybe at Marge. I worked when I got home yesterday, had a drink and dinner out with her. She was in-sistent on seeing me and Vic was away. We talked about her prob-lems mostly—with her husband, son, daughter, stepdaughter, who is "terminal" with breast cancer. Her cells were "atypical." (Why do people always talk to me about cancer? I know why, but I wish they wouldn't.) We walk back to the apartment, I wait while the doorman gets her a taxi and as she gets in, she leans forward and says, "Chin up, Vi, you're doing fine!"

I look at her for a moment, astonished, and then go upstairs and look at myself in the bathroom mirror. Bare light. What did she see? I look fine, I feel fine, my belly hurts, but whose wouldn't, one month post-surgery? I laugh and when Vic comes home, I laugh again when he sees my note to myself, *Chin up,* on the dresser, and explain.

But this morning, when Vic woke up early, I did too, only I kept my eyes closed because I was already angry. I am a little angry at him, ureasonably, because we have agreed that he is to go down to Sarasota with the grandchildren ahead of me, on Friday, since I have to wait to have my shot on Monday. I am a little angry that he wants to take *them,* although I love them, and I think about it. Why? Because they interfere with a fantasy I have of the two of us going off together? But he has a backache, and I have a bellyache, and there is nothing romantic about us. Not now. (I will think about this aspect later. Too painful.) I think some more and suddenly am fearful something will happen to the three of them (I am *very* angry, right?), and then I am truly panic-stricken. Nothing must happen to them, ever, not any of them, especially the grandchildren. I am overwhelmed by the thought that the grandchildren—Kim and Polly—are my own immortality. Not my own daughters, but my grandchildren. I have a sense of their tying me to the earth that is so strong—a sense of continuity that is so shattering—that I am shocked to see what is really behind it: my own inner sense of needing to be at-tached, my feeling that I am slipping away, my *anger,* as Yeats put it speaking of old age, at me, the essential, living, pulsing me be-ing tied to a dying animal. I am not angry at *people,* I see, I am angry at circumstances.

A little at people too, and I feel unable to do anything about it. To say anything, that is. Why? I am afraid of being demanding, complaining, self-serving. (I know. What am I doing now except being demanding, complaining, self-serving?) I feel less whole (today, that is, this angry morning, this morning which is indeed part of chemotherapy because that is what keeps rubbing my nose in the fact that I am less whole). I feel less of a person, less— okay, say it—desirable. I have been aware of this since my first surgery. The scar on my stomach makes me feel impaired. I feel I have to please, rather than be pleased. I feel that Vic is saddled with a second-class wife (I am conscious of my bills, and my not earning money—"You have me as a pet, with big vet bills," I say in jest), and I feel I ought to make it up to him by being as agree-able as I can be. How agreeable that may be, I have no idea—I don't know what living with me is like now. So I woo, instead of expecting to be wooed. His back surgery didn't seem to change the situation much—he doesn't feel second-class. (Not in relation to me anyway—I get glimpses of it in other areas—but I am already an invalid, in a sense, so he isn't imposing on me. I don't know if feel. On this angry morning. This afternoon I probably won't feel any of this is so, he may not feel any of it at all, it's just the way I this way. Or tomorrow. Or, at least if I do, it will be below the surface again.)

To go back to the chemotherapy.

Some of my feeling second-class—i.e., not as strong—is, I suppose, post-surgery. Not connected with chemotherapy. But then what am I saying? Of course it's connected, else I wouldn't have had the surgery in the first place.

I am having a lot of difficulty with semantics. Who am I? Not in the sense the young use the phrase; more accurately, I guess, the question should be, what am I? A cancer patient? I cannot grasp, or accept that. That is why I got so angry at the phrase, "Chin up!" What does she mean? Who does she mean? I look over my shoulder to see whom she is looking at. But if I am getting chemotherapy (whether it is prophylactic or therapeutic is immaterial, it's all semantics, isn't it?), then I *am* a cancer patient. But I don't feel like one, and I don't know if that is denial or not. (I guess that's funny, my not knowing, but I mean it in a psychological sense.)

I feel trapped.

I want to take off. Do something. Travel. Live. Unreasonable, I know. Whether I had had surgery or not—here I go, avoid the word again—I would be exactly where I am now, in the apartment, or in the apartment in Sarasota, or in the house in Mount Kisco, in my goddamn kitchens and closets and bathrooms, right, we are trapped by our things! And Vic has to work. He can't take off anytime he wants. And I don't want to go away alone. I don't even want to go away. I want to work. So nothing is different. I didn't take off before. *But now I know I can't.* Which isn't quite true either. If I wanted to, I could—as I could have before. But I don't want to. Alone. That is, without Vic.

(It's like having an affair. I didn't, I don't want to, but now, I feel that if I wanted to, I couldn't. I have the present, but not the future. Does anyone? Not really. But I know it. Except I don't.)

Still—before I started with this chemotherapy I was getting strong and feeling like myself again, whatever that is (and even that's not true; strong or weak, in the last year, I have always felt "less than," as my introduction pointed out).

Anyway—maybe projecting what I think other people think about me—I feel different, and anything that reminds me of it, I resent. I see, too, that I made a great mistake visiting a friend of mine who died last year. I used to make a point of discussing her illness with her. I thought it was a release for her to be able to talk about it with someone. Chutzpah. Yenta chutzpah. Not to be dignified by the word hubris. You don't want to talk about it. It's only a part of you. A small part. (Whistling in the dark?) You are *you*.

My God, how torn we get! Resent it when people ask how we are, resent it when they don't. ("I'm fine, how else should I be?" "Don't they care? Why don't they call?")

I feel better now. Naturally.

But I'm still trapped.

For the record, Vic just called. "You seemed upset this morning," he says. (I am obviously a delight to live with.) "I was," I say, "but no more." I tell him the above, a smattering anyhow. How wonderful to be able to tell him, as well as friend Royal 440. I feel absolutely great. Now. At 11:30 a.m., Tuesday, February 11.

Week 3. Sitting in Mark's office waiting to see him (I have a ten o'clock appointment so I have to wait—at nine o'clock I am the first one). First thing I think of is my friend Ruth again, the one who asked me if I didn't mind being "experimented with." We saw them last night, and when Vic asked her if she had been doing anything interesting, her first response was: "Well, I just called this friend who has lung cancer, and she is really doing very well." He changed the subject without blinking an eye. I realize that it's all she thinks of around me. It's the way I used to be with blacks, I think—I had to bite my tongue to keep from mentioning Martin Luther King or the March on Washington or—no, not quite true. But it *was* in my mind! I never realized how much I appreciated people who don't mention it, or don't know, or don't ask me how I am, or pamper me. Enough of it.

Kathy asked me if I resent coming here. I never thought about it. I have no choice. (That's why I don't ask what medication I'm getting—it's not up to me.) Now, sitting here, I think I do resent the necessity a little. Still, I am not as afraid before the visit as I used to be. I figure I'm at rock bottom. There's nothing else that can be done for me anyhow. (Yesterday I put away the surgical socks and tried to get myself to throw out the girdle I don't wear anyhow. Christ, I hope I never have to be operated on again! Would I do it? Would I have a choice? Depends, doesn't it? Nonsense, I'd do what I was told.)

I think about Vic's back. In a way, I'm relieved he can't race around. I'm not guilty then about our staying quiet. On the other hand, I feel so dependent on him now—not dependent in a bad way, I depend on him, that's different—when he's not well, I feel insecure.

I let my sister-in-law Edith drive me here today—she's waiting in the car outside—and she is going to take me to the airport. I protested at first, then heard something in her voice, remembered the years I was on call for her, and finally said, "Yes, thank you very much." She said, "My God, chalk one up for me!" What is the line between taking graciously and not imposing?

I think of the novel at home. I got to page 200 yesterday, and I was depressed. If I finish it, what will I do? I've put too much in, I know it, it's two novels really, my editor will probably toss half of it out, but then, will I get a chance to do two books? (Dr. Joffe's joke to Helen after giving her the results of a physical—"Well, don't start any long books.")

I wish my stitch wouldn't hurt, and that my scar wasn't so blatant—then I could forget when I see myself.

All I have to do today is have my shots (Mark doesn't examine me any more, nothing he can do anyhow, I guess, even if he should find something) and go to the airport and then to Sarasota.

The distance from here, in the office, where I'm waiting and writing this, to there, feels so VAST—like crossing Siberia—it's the distance between being a patient and a healthy person. I could cry —it looms so!

I see I still haven't come to grips with my status. Am I a cancer patient, or an "in-case" one? That, too, is a distance as great as the time between Moscow and Irkutsk.

Time. I go into Mark's office, and this visit he has me strip and go through the examining process. So I was wrong. It isn't useless. He skipped the last two times because it was only one week since I had left the hospital.

How am I? Fine, except for the muscle twinge in my stomach. I've gained two more pounds. I weigh more than I have in decades.

I say I'll diet. Mark says, "You'll diet when I tell you." Nice. I'm being managed. Dry mouth? No. Problems? No. No? Well— Am I, or am I not, a cancer patient, or is it semantics?

He gives me a long and careful answer, speaking exactly to my condition: There are some twelve million blood cells being renewed daily in my body (or did he say "billion"?; irrelevant, since it's a metaphor anyway), aside from skin cells, liver cells, etc. All have to be exact, cloned, with one hundred thousand genetic factors taken into consideration. There is a theory that *everyone has cancer cells all the time* which are usually destroyed. In my case, some were destroyed, some got away; the few that didn't get destroyed were found in my biopsy. Chemically, therefore, I have cancer. Clinically, no, since there is no tumor evident which has to be reduced or destroyed. The verdict: uncertainty.

"Like Heisenberg?" I say. Or the nonstandard mathematics I just read about in the *Times.* I am comforted at the thought that uncertainty reigns in such certainties as mathematics and physics, too.

Mark agrees. We agree that the more one knows, the more

one is aware of how much one doesn't know. He mentions something about not bathing in the same river twice; I point out that it is never the same bather either.

End of visit.

Edith takes me to the airport but we stop first to eat, for as usual I have no nausea, simply a ravenous appetite. Also, exactly an hour after the shots, I feel a flush. Period.

At 2:15 p.m. I am on the plane. A healthy person. At six p.m. I am at the apartment with Vic and the kids, and I go down to swim. I swim slowly at first, but I look up at the blue sky and see the gulls dipping, and all I can think is, "What a miracle!" Six weeks ago, I swam and looked up and wished for—what? Exactly this—to be able to swim and see the blue sky and the gulls dipping.

By the next day I am swimming as well—or as badly—as ever.

Among the books Vic has taken from the library is one called *Widow*. I assume he has taken it out for me, so I read it. I go down to the pool and tell him it was a very good book. He agrees. It turns out that he read it, too. I look at him, a little taken aback. So he, too, must have an *idée fixe*. I recall how Lynn Caine says she regrets that they never talked about their fears. We take a walk on the beach and I say tentatively, "You're not worried about me, are you?" "Of course not," he says, and I laugh. "Some question! How else can you answer?" We walk some more, and I begin. "I was wondering whether or not I was really a cancer patient, so I asked Mark. And do you know what he said? There are twelve million blood cells . . ."

I find an article by L. E. Sissman in an *Atlantic* I left in the apartment last time. It is about chemotherapy, which didn't much interest me at the time. He has Hodgkin's disease and describes the chemotherapy—eighteen months of it—he had for a third bout. Brief nausea only in the late afternoon of the day of injection.

Little hair loss. (I have a bit on my brush, I think—but who knows? I always did before.) He says the first six months of treatment "seemed a breeze," but the second took a toll. It was "spirit-killing," the cyclic medical routine, that is. He dreads the "prolonged prick of an I.V. needle feeling its way into a vein." A good piece. Specific. Nothing phony about it. I file it, not that I feel that way—yet, but I may want some company someday.

My horoscope in *Vogue:* "My advice—remember that miracles have a habit of happening to those who believe in them."

Margit—who had worked for us for sixteen years and has no one but us essentially—calls. She has an infection in her breast. The doctor wants to hospitalize her, she is going to wait until she gets back. (She is on her first vacation in years—in Florida.) I am angry. Everything happens to her. (I forget about me.) Also—let this cup pass, O Lord. It sours the rest of the few days, and the next two weeks too. I am scared for her, resentful at the burden, ashamed at being resentful, very conscious of what I have put people through around me. And then we have the day of surgery—I go down early, go with her to the operating room, wait through the recovery room, the surgeon forgets to tell me she's all right, I don't know until she's actually down, and all I can think of is "My God, what I have put them all through!" But what can I do? What could I do?

Jan has a sort of surprise birthday party for me. I am very touched, not sure I want being sixty to be celebrated (Vic has a thing about birthdays anyhow), but also sure that any birthday now *should* be celebrated. So I get dressed up, put on *all* my jewelry, and am stunned to catch a fleeting thought, "It's all right to wear everything I have. No one will begrudge it to me now."

Forgot about Polly's fall from the diving board and her stitches. I was very shaken in the emergency room and later. (Vic and I took the kids out to dinner afterward and I had two drinks in a row.) My tolerance for everything seems much lower these days. Or am I simply freer to acknowledge my fears, tiredness, sense of put-uponnesses, etc.? I don't know.

Series 2

March 10. I do think I'm not as worried about seeing Mark as I used to be. But I did have an anxiety dream Saturday night— I was trying to register for college, ended up in a mass auditorium, like the old Albee Building, last seat in the last row, couldn't get a catalogue, didn't know what courses to take, and every English course I could find was so inferior I wanted to say, "But I can teach this better."

Sunday night I had another anxiety dream (awhile back it was about being eighteen again, having to go on dates, find a man), and this time I was a little child. I was buying baby lotions, creams, etc., in a shopping center, and I was also my mother or sister, helping me, and it was all very confusing.

The anxiety dreams are all of starting life all over again, and they always seem to end with a kind of relieved statement that I can't, I'm going to die, I've been through it already.

I sleep fitfully after that. Wake up with a remark: "I am leaving the world of the whole!"

I think I am a little nervous because I am going to drive to Mark's and back. I think of taking a plastic bag in case I have to throw up but I forget to. I have a heavy feeling waiting in the office this time. Not fear of what will be found, just a kind of pervasive sense of doom.

We talk of how difficult it is to express oneself truly (because I haven't given him any of this yet), and I am examined. I have gained more weight. Everyone commented on how well I look—I begin to feel as if maybe I am on cortisone. I ask Mark if it is the medicine, and he says, yes, he thinks it is. Shall I diet? No. He also asks me to go to the lab to be checked on Friday, a request very simple to honor, but one which depresses me again.

For the first time I feel that this is for real. It is going to go on and on and on. It's like having a baby. First time, the labor pains are fascinating. You can't wait to see what will happen next. (Surgery too; in fact, all processes.) Second time, not so fascinating. You know. Maybe the same thing with these treatments. Sissman's cyclical depression? Am I feeling what I *think* I should feel?

I drive home and as I near the garage I am very pleased. No problem at all. I fill the prescription and feel a kind of rash on my face. The flush, I guess. It subsides.

I am starved. Not only that. I eat four candies at lunch: (a) because they are here, which is rare for this house; (b) because I feel I want to comfort myself (never before with food); and (c) if it is the shots, not food, that make me fat, what difference does it make?

Day 2. I took my pills this morning as casually as if they were vitamins.

Friday I had to go to the lab to have my blood count and such tested.

Thursday night I had anxiety dreams, fleeting, but enough to wake me each hour on the hour. Why? I'm not sure, except that the last time I woke up, I was angry. I tried to figure out what was going on, but all I could come up with was that the lab was ugly—a small warren of shabby apartment rooms off Madison Avenue with a dusty waiting room about the size of a subway lavatory.

I stopped at the lab on the way to the country. It took me longer to find a garage in which to park (at two dollars for fifteen minutes!) than to have my blood taken.

And when I left, I realized why I had been uneasy and angry. The young Chinese girl who took my blood this time was quick and, if not friendly, neutral. But the aide who took care of me at my last visit, which was my first there, radiated hostility. I don't know why, she just did. Was I, perhaps, exaggerating her lack of interest? Did I expect some fellow feeling because of what she was deciphering—a cancer follow-up? Was I queasy about her knowing what I was there for? (I had tried, vainly, to have my prescription for the fifteen little white chemotherapy pills filled at Montefiore earlier in the week; for some reason I didn't want my druggist to see that I was taking them. But I had to have him fill the prescription anyway; he, too, was noncommittal, although last time I got something—toothpaste, I think it was—he looked at me and said, "Are you feeling all right, Mrs. Weingarten?" I wondered what he meant. We don't use a druggist in the city much. He wouldn't have known anything about my medical history. All we've gotten from him are antibiotics and Valium.)

I go into my lab reaction because I think there are two factors at work here.

First, I am accustomed, I am afraid, to the kind of medical care few people get—personal, interested, caring. And, to be truthful, I am accustomed to thinking of myself as "special." The offhand lab puts my nose out of joint.

Second, and more pertinent maybe, I feel about cancer deep down the way people used to feel about "consumption" (or syphilis). I am ashamed of having it (if indeed I do ☺).*

In a conversation with my friend Ellen (also receiving chemotherapy) today, in which she reported that someone we know is back in the hospital: "They had to take him off chemotherapy. It's all experimental anyway, you know."

She goes on to say that she is one who asks many questions of her doctors, then asks me what drugs I am getting. I tell her I don't know, and then forthrightly I tell her I don't ask because I don't want to know. "I don't want to pick up a newspaper and read of the reactions I am supposed to be getting, and don't." Well! So that's why I keep my peace! Good for me. That makes sense.

Speaking of reactions, Mark asked me last time if I had a

* The face is a sign of embarrassment, right?

"dry mouth." Would a dry "back of the throat" count? If so, I do.
A little.

Passover. I read a headline in the *Times* about a "cancer cure
breakthrough." (One-day wonder it turns out to be. I see no
reference to it at any other time, don't even remember what it
was.) I get very excited and realize how wonderful it would be if
indeed a cure was found. (Later in the month I read about
Einstein Medical Center getting a cancer research grant and one of
the doctors mentions the "thirty diseases that are cancer." Reassuring somehow. Like Joey Mandelbaum years ago saying fever
can mean a hundred different ailments.)

Vic says Mark is delighted about how well I am doing. My
reaction—why shouldn't I do well? What is there for me to do
well about? (I know now—my reaction to the chemotherapy. At
least I suppose so.) I mention my weight, but he says Mark is
pleased about that. (Why? If it is the medicine that is doing it? I
suppose if it weren't taking, and I were ill, I would be losing. So
it *is* something.)

Anyway I am both pleased and scared at the report. Evil eye
again? I should go back to my advice to Edna O'Brien. What kind
of Being would it be if it punished for hope? And if there is no
Being, why so scared of what you think?

I finish the first draft of the novel (really the first of many
drafts) and allow myself to be happy about it. I even call Michael
to tell him. Vic brings champagne. I have a fleeting thought: "I
can die now."

(Note: Right after Mark told Vic I was fine, I got such a
pain on the top part of my scar, I can't do any exercises. Now, as I
write, the scar in my right shoulder feels raw.)

Series 2 is finished, and we go to Sarasota. My daughter Kathy
too, for the weekend.

First morning on the beach I see a baby. Right away I think of Kathy because we have talked the night before about the timing of her pregnancy-to-be. (That makes me uneasy too. They have to have it timed so exactly—to coincide with Hilary's second residency year and the end of her teaching year, so he can be with the infant part-time and she doesn't disappoint her students.) Will I be around for the as-yet-unconceived infant? Not so much for my sake, but for hers. Rituals are very important to her.

Well, I'm getting chemotherapy. That ought to keep me going. I think of the Le Shan piece I read on the plane coming down. He does faith-healing by thinking of the tumor and visualizing it getting smaller. I walk farther down the beach and think of a faintly scarred place inside my colon and try to think of it shrinking. I determine to keep fighting it off. I'm happy. Do happy people die of cancer? Must be some people who are happy who can't fight it off. I think of what Dr. Gleidman said, "If it comes back, we'll cut it out." Simple. Okay, one more time. For Kathy. Is any of this real to me? No. I'm doing what Kathy does—trying to think of eventualities and solve them in my mind. Or rather, Kathy does what I have done all my life. Does it help? I don't know. I don't think I actually expected any of the major traumas that happened—or if I did, they didn't come or affect us as I had expected.

I told Kathy that I had told Irene, a friend we saw at the theater. "So you told her of the fly in the ointment, right?" is Kathy's comment. Interesting. In that case, I am using the cancer as a talisman. As long as I have that, I am exempt from everything else. The dues have been paid. Does a little cancer exempt you from more cancer? Why not?

Sex—just fine. Even the scar doesn't seem to mean much, although I do pull up the sheet afterwards. But I forget during. As a matter of fact, my heaviness seems to make me more sensual. (Is there testosterone in the medication? I'm confused here. If it is given to sex prisoners—that is, Depo- something is—to make them less perverse, why should it make me heterosexually more aroused? Or am I? I really can't tell. I guess I'm essentially the same.)

My weight—I seem to eat a lot. Pills? Would I be fat even if I didn't eat so much? My body feels very strange to me. I am used to feeling light and spare. Now I feel as if I am inhabiting a stranger—someone broad, chunky, solid. Too thin is less strange to me than too fat. Still I look better, in my face anyway, and I pull my shirts over my pants to disguise the lack of waistline, and so far I seem to be getting away with it publicly.

Vic keeps acting—or at least, has the grace to let me think he is—as if my weight gain is a great feat on my part which makes me look wonderful.

Sign of optimism—I buy a new bathing suit.

Vic has trouble finding a tennis partner. The couple he plays with finds a couple to play with, leaving him without a game. I start to say what I would usually say: "Your next wife will be a tennis player," but this time I don't go on with it.

I walk down the beach, thinking of how I react to Mark's comments about my condition. If he says I'm doing fine, I worry (well, see what happened last November). If he doesn't, I worry even more.

We have come to Sarasota each time I finished a series of treatments. It's been wonderful because as soon as I get here I begin to swim, and my body feels more like its old self. I also feel well. It all seems fairly far away.

This time I am uneasy about leaving. We aren't coming back until next season, unless we sell the place, in which case we'll have to come down to close it and not come at all next season. (Which I hope. Although there is a sense of finality about all our trying to sell—again, I'm torn. I want to sell Sarasota and the Mount Kisco house in order to be *free* to do things I would find more interesting—travel, rent somewhere else, get a little apartment maybe, and of course, mostly for Vic to be free of all the expense and responsibility. On the other hand, there is a sense of trying to put my affairs in order, a finality, a getting rid of old clothes, objects, etc., that otherwise the kids would have to do.)

So I am scared. Is this the last time? Not for the proper reason—a sale—but because I might be sick.

I listen to the ocean in the morning. I think that if I were ill, I would like to lie and listen to it. (There is a sound machine I read about that does just that—gives you white sound and the sound of the sea—it would be pleasant, wouldn't it, to cease upon the midnight with no pain listening to the sea? *With no pain.* Ah, there's the rub. I am suddenly terrified of dying. It feels as if it is for the first time, but it's probably not.)

I pack mentally and close out everything that is personal in the apartment.

My mind is making me uncomfortable so I pick up *The Outermost House,* which is on my bedside table. Beston says: "For a moment of night we have a glimpse of ourselves and of our world islanded in its stream of stars—pilgrims of mortality, voyaging between horizons across eternal seas of space and time."

Comforting in the abstract.

But I remember how the concept scared hell out of me after my first surgery, picking up a science magazine in the anteroom of the nuclear medicine section and seeing a picture of our planet in the universe and thinking of myself as a dot in an eternity of space . . . I didn't want to be a dot, I wanted to be ME, big as life (and now, bigger by the minute).

Series 3

April 15. First time at journal in a month—a good sign. I've been too busy with the book (but I've taken notes).

I come out of the bedroom at 8:15 deciding I'd better type this and find the machine open and ready for use—a good omen for the day. I feel better.

This has been an edgy twenty-four hours, all in my head. Left for the bus yesterday at eight a.m., Vic taking me and waiting in the car at the bus stop—nice. I got to Mark's office in half an hour, waited an hour and a half (I have to get him some magazines other than ancient *Reader's Digests*). Nothing to say to him really—still another good sign—except I'm fat, which I'll continue to be, and a bit hirsute, and hoarse, all symptoms. So. Shall I diet? No. I decide to ask at least how long. "I don't want to put you on the spot but is it open-ended?" Quickly he says he doesn't know—same drugs this time, he's very pleased, but who knows? As I figured. I imagine it'll be a year or two, maybe spaced a little more. Ellen says all my life. Who knows what that means, either? Anyway shall I buy pants to last through summer? At least six months—oh, yes. In the office I say I've not worked on the journal, too busy. He says that's the best medicine, to be busy, and then says something about psychiatrists not being helpful (I think I said something about not having brooded—but do I? I was just talking really, to have something to say). I tell him about reading about terminal illness and how to take it, but say I'm really more chronic, although no pain, he says, yes, and so on . . .

Long wait for pills. Home by two. A really wasted morning, almost day. Too tired to write. Out to dinner with Vic. Just lovely. But—here the edgy part—I had picked up *New York* magazine, and there is a story that Depo-Provera (the drug Ellen gets) is used to cut sex drive of criminals. Am I getting it? Does it work the same way with women? I had made a note to write about sex yesterday—about how good mine (ours) is—is it pills? Not related? Am I getting that drug? Does it—will it—have effect? Proves again that I really shouldn't know the name of my medication—too iffy a business—so much for that.

I wake up this morning thinking about Depo-, because for once, having gone to bed early and slept hard, I don't feel anything physical at all. Want to read paper, nothing else. Drug? (I know this is funny, but that's how it goes.) Get paper. Page 1. Fredric March dead of cancer. Ugh. Turn on TV. Breast cancer commercial. Honestly. Turn to paper. Hear Barbara Walters mention March's death, then she says a friend of ours just died last night and tells about Edith Vanocur and her gallant fight. "We all hoped she was going to make it, but the end was inevitable."

I forget. Talked to my sister Jean after Dad asked when I was coming down to Florida. I was very hoarse. Explained. Also the weight. Suddenly realized I was giving untrue impression— I'm *not* all that affected. She said she wished I had Christian Science. Was going to pray harder. I have to call her more often. But I wish my father would stop nudging me to come down. I think I'll tell him.

I go in and take my three little pills.

I hope this is it for the day.

Vic hugs me a couple of times when he says goodbye. I must be so hard to live with. What would I do if it were reversed? (Well, Kathy said his cholesterol puts him in the 70 percent risk bracket, but that has no reality to me. Maybe I don't for him either.)

Monday, April 21. Little foxes to report. Thyroid palpable. Right hand numb at night. Feeling pre-menstrual. Sense that the poisons are taking hold, for good, or for ill. Mark says bloods are stable, except for platelets, "which we watch very carefully." Don't ask him what he means. He gives me the same complete checkup as last week. Why every week? (Because I complained—in this journal—that he wasn't doing it every week?)

Weight—130½. No gain this week. I'm in new 12 and 14 pants, but also oddly fit into a few of my eights. Waistline isn't very different. Just fat pads.

For the first time, nothing to talk about with Mark. I have the sense he is keeping something from me. Paranoia? But he did check my reflexes this time. Didn't ask why. Probably the numbness is the reason.

I think, should I mention Depo-Provera article? Also sex, It's fine—decide not to. Don't want to stir up sleeping dogs.

I see Gleidman. He is pleased with my stomach muscles, says exercise won't do anything about fat, anyhow fat is good—many people on chemotherapy get thin. "You don't need a doctor," he says. But in the office, he tells me to come back in three or four months. "I'm here. I don't expect anything, but that's the way I function. Also, better have a barium enema in the fall. No reason, that's the way I do it." He's right, and I should feel safe, but I don't. I feel scared already of the fall. I put it down in my book for October instead of September. (This morning I fantasized asking Mark to put off tests to January instead of in November when I assume they come due again—as usual, the gun is jumped on me.) We talk for once—I tell about Crile article on excessive surgery. He says Crile hated his father, a super surgeon. I tell him about rectal surgery instead of burning—(no connection with me, of course). He says it's easy to do a little operation, but maybe you don't cure the patient. I have fantasy of how much surgery I would allow if . . . I have fantasy discussion with him and he understands. (He did, in fact, tell me that he had never had surgery and became a surgeon because he was "scared—that's why surgeons become surgeons." Would he understand? Would he let a knife slip? Break his record for the "good" of the patient? Never.)

Lunch with Alice. Among other things she talks of her brother's heart illness and how "I went into a depression after he left, kept thinking of death and illness." I look at her. "You have to live as if," I say, and wonder who is kidding whom.

Am I sick? I still keep looking over my shoulder. Who are they saying is "doing well"? Who are they pleased is "fat"? Who do they think has to be "checked"? Not me. I don't know about you, bud, I'm okay.

Funny thing is I think I am okay. Both ways.

I come home, see hair on the side of my face, am appalled. First time. How long have I had it? I get angry for a second. How

can Mark do this to me? I take it off. Reflect on the minor cour-
ages this all needs—like the woman who took as gallantry putting
on lipstick every morning. Well, the hair remover is one. (I had to
do it on my lip before.) So is the lubricating cream. Very little
foxes. IF THIS IS ALL . . .

I think Gleidman actually saw me as a person today. Or I
saw him. Mention that I finished book. (I'm really pleased, I
realize.) "Oh, you write? I didn't know what you did." Tell about
the three novels. Mention Knopf. He is duly impressed. But signifi-
cantly—"What you write now is different, I'll bet—I want to see
what you wrote before the first operation." I like that. So he does
see the person for the scar.

We talked about what surgery does for people. I think
it—the cancer—gave me a new lease (in a way). Does surgery do
it for most? He says yes, "no matter how it comes out." "They've
brooded about it, they're relieved, at first they're tired—then they
get better and have a burst of energy," and "each time they're reassured, the burst continues." He says I looked wan before, as
though I was tense about something, and I am no more. Is that
possible? I thought that particular tenseness had stopped. Maybe
not. But I don't think I am tense now.

I hope the hair isn't the start of a line of unpleasantnesses.

If I were alone, I would not be afraid. Two reasons. I
wouldn't care what happened to me. I wouldn't worry about being
a bother. The last is the main thing that troubles me always. No
matter how I try to circumvent it—fantasy of the great life Vic will
have after; it is worth paying for, think of Michael and others.
Still do not know how I could bear it. Or a colostomy. Again, in
re Vic.

Cut it out.

The only life you have is your own.

.   .

April 24. Visit to Dr. Rifkin, my GP. Hilarious. "You look marvelous, blooming." Big embrace. He takes my blood pressure. "Thank God." Listens to my heart. "Thank God." Feels thyroid. "Too soft." Period. Nurse does EKG. "We'll compare this one with the old one, in case, God forbid, there is any change." In the office, he says I'm fine except for the thyroid. (Is that why the weight?) Ear, nose, and throat perfect. Except that he didn't look at any of them. "See me in three months." Why?

I buy some size-12 pants and a too-expensive skirt from Micmac. Usual dialogue with myself. Why not?

Miriam calls. Didn't hear from me. Worried about effects of chemotherapy. Pleased, and a little uneasy. What effects should I have?

See my friend Jean. She met the Silvers. They told her. Are you getting chemotherapy? Yes. "Can't be much. You look fine."

At night I am tired. (I have been working all day and into the evening on the ms.) Not interested in sex. The medication? Am I getting Depo- etc.? On the other hand, why so interested before? Better in a.m. But thought flashes all the same.

Do people with bad hearts flinch every time they read obits? EVERYBODY dies of it. William Alanson White leaflet describes last days of Janet Rioch—her gallantry in the face of suffering. Well, for Christ's sake, what did you expect? *Do* you expect? (I don't like this candid journal. Suddenly I remember that Mark is going away at the end of August—a good omen, I thought in the office, he can leave me. On the other hand, if the shots come then . . . I want to go to China, to Alaska, anywhere. I'll take my bottles with me.)

I take out a new ream of paper—last one. Is it my last? Please God.

. .

April 25. No sweat at all. I go to the lab for the usual and think of Sissman's remark that it becomes increasingly difficult to maintain the therapy. Not really. But time has stretched for me, instead of flying. It feels like many months, but it is only—I keep counting—three. Less than, actually. I have come so far in these three months. I feel—knock wood—so strong. It seems to me that inside of a month, it's as though the whole thing wasn't, but maybe I'm remembering wrong.

I am still fearful about giving up the book. Exactly like having a baby. The last days you can't wait, and you are also frightened. No, it's different. The reason you are scared then is that you *will* have something to fill your days; now it's the reverse. Plus the subliminal fear—will this be the last? Will I ever see it? I want to show people the ms. I keep thinking of ironies—this will be the "good one," as my agent, Anne, said in her letter, and I won't know it. Nonsense. Only a year. I'll be around, one way or the other.

Driving up to the country it struck me that this is a special journal. In the first place it is open-ended. I shan't end it, life will. Also, I am a very special person (anyone like me is). Superhuman in this sense—the mark of being human is knowing you will die. True of anyone, but in this case, more so. Also, the other mark is speech, communicating, writing down. True here, too.

Shoulder hurts, stomach hurts—probably the rain (also that the latter is only three months). Poor Vic. We spare each other our worries; what's the use of saying the same thing over and over? Anyway if I'm busy, I don't brood. So I brood about whether I am going to be busy!

April 26. I am now the mother of a thirty-two-year-old.

. .

"Nothing happens to any man that he is not formed by nature to bear." Marcus Aurelius.

"For that which is born death is certain, and/or the dead, birth is certain. Therefore grieve not over that which is unavoidable." Bhagavad-Gita.

Today. Saturday. Woke up at seven with my right hand tingling and numb. So reminded. Am frightened, too. Realize that I was so lucky to have come out of the hospital in the middle of work—really, a week or so later I was at the typewriter. But there is a price. *Now* I am confronting it.

But I shall not be frightened, I think. For everything a season. This is the time to make peace with it again, to be empty and to fill up.

Vic reaches out. I worry. How can I respond when in my head . . . will I ever again? But I stroke, we pat . . . and an explosion. I don't have to worry. And I feel fine.

In the shower I think of my Aunt Peggy. And a book begins to take shape. I know all about her now. A lot more anyhow. The pain of being deserted, and alone (and keeping her love intact). The terrors of living with illness (hers was painful, debilitating, but more open-ended)—she plans to end it when the time comes —but it never does. Even in the hospital there was something to live for: "The nurses say I'm a sight for sore eyes," as indeed she was. It falls into place. A way of saying what I have to say.

From St. Augustine: "Give me chastity and continency, but not yet."

"Love, and do what you will." (Love God?)

Last words of Queen Elizabeth I "All my possessions for a moment of time."

"O ye Whales, and all that move in the water." Book of Common Prayer.

"Wonders are many, and none is more wonderful than man." Sophocles, *Antigone.*

. .

April 28. Last day of shots for Series 3.

I go up to the Bronx. Careful exam about the breasts. Lifts legs (nerve damage?) Takes platelet count (why?). But no vaginal, or rectal (had each week in past). How am I doing? Who knows? Gained half a pound more at least.

We talk about historical novels—Josephine Tey. My God, Mark knows a lot about English history. It makes up for the County Medical Society poster in the waiting room (not his, of course).

Not much to say—except I need a barium enema in June! Terrifies me.

On the way down I realize I am angry again. Trapped. No exit. Am I worse off than a Vietnam refugee? Poor old person? Is it the worst? In theory maybe. Actually, not at all, because, so far, it is only in theory. But the anger, and the feeling of being trapped persists. I have to live it out. I am afraid of being afraid, believe I have to think positive thoughts. On the other hand I can't fool myself, can I? Can't say, be positive, or, I am positive, when I'm not. I realize this too will pass . . .

Talked to Vic about it last night. I say my tolerance is very low, which is true. I am jealous of my time, I really care only about him and me and the kids and who else?—Helen maybe. Terrible—or is it? It's fact (not so different from before—I wasn't mad for most of my friends or to be a good daughter—I'm just more honest about it now, at least my body is). My face looks exhausted. I wonder how I look to others? The pictures Vic took are good, but the closeup of my face looks lined. Anyhow I told him I was having a time adjusting to the end of the book—again, as usual, only more so. I have a problem about how much to say to him. If I don't share I set up a wall, but I don't want to worry him because my moods *do* change, *and* I don't want him to look at me differently.

Anyhow back to today. As I allow the anger to surface it

dribbles out. It is sunny and I like driving down and I say I will do one pleasant thing a day from now on. I call Vic and he asks me to lunch. I am delighted, and we have a lovely lunch with wine, go to UN.—I walk home, market—nicely dizzy—and feel fine. The day's nice thing. I am lucky.

I think while waiting at the Bibliothèque (outside looking at the UN) that maybe having cancer is better than a heart attack—you literally get time as a gift. It is the salt that gives savor—minus pain, disfigurement, disgust. In the mind, it is as enhancing as it is frightening (keep thinking that if Vic died I wouldn't mind, it's the fear of burdening him that gets me). But death is a heavy price for him to pay to escape it, so maybe I should keep holding on to that: the only way to escape the pain of a loved one's death (but I don't think of myself as the loved one, only as a burden) is to die first. Sudden is a shock, drawn out is awful, but relieves you of guilt, I guess. Oh, shit—you take care of that one, God.

April 30. I walk up Fifth Avenue to return the faith-healing books to Judy Tobias's doorman. I pass Temple Emanu-El. It is a beautiful sunny afternoon. I decide I will go in and pray. Make a wish. But what wish? From general to particular. I settle on nothing to be found in the June barium enema. But the temple is closed. I go to the side entrance at Sixty-fifth Street, walk into the chapel, stand there for a moment, feel like an idiot. How can I possibly pray? Especially in a world so fraught that churches have to be locked against intruders.

(All this tentative prayer, evil eye stuff, wondering whether I should take up Zen—I read in the *Times* Sunday that Peter Matthiessen, author of *Far Tortuga,* took up Zen together with his "late" wife to stand the strain of her terminal illness. All of this unnerves me. This morning, though, I read in a story about amulets, potions, etc., at the Jewish Museum that magic can be considered either as superstition or an acknowledgment of helplessness in the face of the mystery. Certainly the last is valid, considering that we don't even know the why's of what I am being treated for, or have any certainty about the means.)

Only three months since surgery. I keep forgetting. I feel so normal that when tiredness suddenly hits me, it's a shock.

May Day. What would I do if Vic didn't keep saying I have a great figure? It's as if I had something to do with it, something good, instead of . . . But it's very reassuring.

I realize the date. Barium enema in June. I'm scared. Better to have it early so I have the summer. If they find something it will be little. But I can't have surgery every few months. On the other hand, they didn't take out anything last time, so it would really date back to a year ago last February. I note only because the ramifications of the mind are incredible. Making good out of bad! Last night I thought a breast cancer isn't so bad, after all, it's outside of you! Good God!

I dream, the first non-ill dream, I think. I'm with Vic at dinner, a lovely place, a lovely time. I say I want to pay—he argues—I insist—finally gives in angrily. "Thanks a lot"—I really didn't mean it—why did I do it? Apologetic—guilty—tell myself to remember next time, was acting nonsexual. (Non-ill dream?)

I am interviewing an old general or somebody. He's in pink crepe de chine sheets, blue silk pj's—good-looking, but drawn. Then he's dark-haired, sleek, and dressed. The point being to imply there's been a relationship. I (very *Vogue* glamorous) say—well, I've had one or two lovers, but . . .

What did the dreams mean?

This is the jerkiest journal of all time. Meanwhile Vietnam falls.

May 2. Vic wakes up, as usual, before seven, and goes out to read the paper. I wake up too, and begin the morning fight with the devils. Pure panic. I realize that I have been thinking of the barium enema since a week ago Monday, when Gleidman suggested it. Mark's putting it up closer made it even scarier. Why?

I guess I thought of chemotherapy as a talisman—if I have it, I don't have to worry. But to have to check every six months even so. It will come when my father is here. Added worry. Go through usual—if it is anything, it will be small, etc.

Denial still continues. If chemotherapy takes care of everything, why the careful physicals? Why Rifkin? The mind is a— what kind of place? I remember—heaven and hell, but what else? —a place of its own? Anyway.

And why am I so frightened? Of bothering Vic. Always. Always have to go through the process. He'll be okay, if—only way for him to avoid it is to be sick himself. But that, of course, is not true. Doesn't have to be either/or. I can be okay too.

The thing that I fear is fear itself.

Same thing happened to me last year, about the same time. It will pass. Actually it has passed, for today. I write it to be truthful, but making beds, finding the *Masterwork Hour* (the days' joys— finding WNYC has music, and UHF all the Channel 13's I miss), having the typewriter, have erased *it* for now.

What kills me (hah!) is that I waste the *good* time worrying? Psychiatry? I don't think it would help. I have reality to cope with. I'll manage. I do. (Fantasy while showering. Book comes out, *Times* gives great review, all my work re-evaluated because Knopf told them I was terminal. Neat way to do it! Still I am something. Four novels since I was—how old? Copyright of *Mrs. Beneker* is '67—eight years—starting at fifty-two. I'm a story, but no one knows it fortunately. I'd hate to be famous because I'm so old.)

Odd notes (gathering up the minutiae).

Just went over my notes for this journal—find I have a lot— so even here I am lucky. I can train the maggots in the wound. (What an image! But then the next thing I think of is Nehru in prison playing with the mongoose in his cell. In our terms, a mongoose is like a rat, isn't it?)

—Lunch with my friend Janet. We manage this afternoon (as we will in afternoons to come) not to mention our secret bond —my surgery, her mastectomy. But I talk about buying my daughter Jan a birthday present, and she tells how she was offered a Gucci bag—"it lasts forever"—and refused—"because I won't." We go to see the Scythian gold at the Met, and I realize their ornaments and saddle blankets are their Gucci bags. Worthwhile? Absolutely.

—Vic sees a story in the *Times* about facials. Suggests I have one. Why not, I think. I have one. As I suspected, silly. I can't stand lying there in the dark for an hour, being fussed over. But it is one of the new self-indulgences. I think of my lab and medical bills per week and decide it amounts to no more than if I were seeing a psychiatrist. I mention this to Jan and her response is, "Getting treatment for cancer is not like seeing a psychiatrist." Or getting a facial? "Treatment for cancer?" I think. But that's what it is, isn't it? Life and death. No choice. But still I refuse to face it.

—My sister Jean on the phone: "Dad keeps asking me what's the matter with you, but I can't use the word. I pray for you. I tell myself that you are taking the medication for the doctor, not for yourself." The family habit of denial is unshakable. I have told my father, many times.

—When I show Bob Gottlieb (my editor at Knopf) the book, he says, "Great stuff about your father. Maybe you want to save it for another book, don't throw it away here." But I can't. I've put everything into it. I don't feel I can save any material. Dad will have to forgive me for not waiting until he is gone to write about him. I don't feel open-ended about time. I want people to read it now, those I care about, that is. I want to hand out the manuscript! But it's not a frightening thought, it's freeing. (Here, too, things are mixed. Writers, cancer or not, generally don't hold back. Mailer, Roth, Jong, all of them, they let it out. But then they're young. Or were. So what it has done for me is allow me to do what I should have done all along.)

—I look up *Of Lena Geyer* to get a sense of style to parody

for one of the little novels in the book. Discover what I did not
pay any attention to when I read it years ago. Lena Geyer died of
cancer, devastatingly. I read the chapters with horror. Such agony!
I look up the date of copyright—1936. Forty years ago! I trust
things are different. Besides it's inaccurate medically. Her cancer is
laid to damage of her cervix in childbirth. Doesn't seem possible.

May 7. Almost a week since I was at this journal, but I've
been taking notes. I shall have to go back and recapitulate a little,
but it's interesting to see where I am.

I handed in the book (complete except for Gottlieb's going
over it) yesterday. I am not as depressed as I was last week when it
became apparent it was finished. I kept spreading it out, reading it
over and over again, polishing—a good thing, because I found all
kinds of minor dissonances, but my motivation was really not to
let go. I always feel scared when I finish a book (funny, to be saying always—but truth to tell, there are eight now—okay, four—
the four nonfiction ones don't count the same way), but this time
it's a little different. Partly because I really don't know what I am
going to write next (but I never did). Partly because it is so important for me to have something going on now (I think that was
what saved me when I got out of the hospital in January—I had
work to pick up on right away). But most of all because of all the
unknowns. Will I see it published? (Next spring.) How will I
feel then? (Will I be another Cornelius Ryan?) Will they push it
(in part because)? How will I feel about that? Diffident if they
do, angry if they don't. Also, a whole lot of me went into it. I can't
retreat any more—write what Gottlieb calls "cutesy"—I can only
write from my gut now. But what I have to write about now is, in
a way, unwritable. Except here.

This, of course, is my next book. But this, too, has a strange-
ness about it. Because I can't really finish it. Or if I do, it will
really be the last. Maybe not. But it can't be published unless there
is something "terminal"; those are the people who talk freely—

and I'm not that, except philosophically. (Okay, here we go again. I am as terminal as anyone, even an infant born this minute, but I am a little more terminal, even though I am not as terminal, say, as anyone with a nonoperable tumor. Shit, to borrow a phrase from an upcoming great novel, entitled, so far, *Half a Marriage.* I'm like Captain Queeg on the subject, rolling my two little balls in my hand—in one way, I am; in another, I'm not. Well, maybe it's true. I'm not being evasive, I'm just acknowledging fact.)

While we're on the subject, I am very pleased about the book. Pleased to have written it. Sure, Jacqueline Susann did it, with no one knowing, but that was brave, too. I don't mean I feel brave. I don't. But I acknowledge that it is something to have made of the two pains of Vic's leaving me and the first surgery something positive and enriching—and good. It *is* a good book— and a love story. I hope Vic realizes that. A true one, too.

Just setting the scene. Now back to where I left off. I hope I dated my notes.

Erik Erikson in last Sunday's *Times* book review (quoted at any rate): "So, it is true, I had to try and make a style out of marginality and a concept out of identity confusion. But I also have learned from life histories that everything that is new and worth saying (or worth saying in a new way) has a highly personal aspect. The question is only whether it is also generally significant for one's contemporaries. That I must let you judge."

I get more first-person every day. The above would be my justification. (I believe it implicitly, of course.)

I am dithering now. I just read some clippings I had included in my note folder. The one that upset me most was an article in *Woman's Day* by Eda Le Shan about the work of her husband, Lawrence. (I actually stole it from the National Airlines copy— my guilt is assuaged because the article says cancer patients are usually "too good," "suppress anger," "conform," etc. I am making progress, then.) I shall go into the issues it raises at another time. What is scary is how in so many ways I conform to the "predicted" cancer patient pattern. What is not scary is that, in that case, I also now conform to the pattern of those who will lick it—for a while anyway. (That, as Kathy and I individually decided, is the catch-22 of thinking cancer is emotionally induced. If you decide it isn't—and Mark's theory of its being a long time developing would indicate not, although, on second thought, maybe not, I'm the same person now I was then, or rather, long ago I was the kind of person I am now, probably more so in the harmful ways—anyway, if you decide it isn't, then you can't assume that right thoughts, living, etc., will help.)

Still, I'll get back to the clippings. Now, some catching up. (I did date my notes except for one about the "lettuce washer." Very significant, that. I don't buy objects for the house. Wouldn't have before, probably. I have so many things. But Jan and Kathy both have special lettuce washers they say are great. I have bought one. A testament of faith, even more than the spring pants I bought, and the dress. The latter were essential if I was to get out of the house or go to the weddings. But the lettuce washer! Sign of life going on. I love it. So much so that now I am brooding over whether I ought to get one for Mount Kisco. I think not. I'll take it with me. Have lettuce washer, will travel.)

While I'm on the subject—the furrier wanted to mend my shabby fur jacket, cost $150. "It will last a lifetime," he said. I agreed, then had second thoughts. The "last a lifetime" was tempting fate and wasteful. I don't even know if I'll use it next winter. (Finger crossing? I really think I will.) Also, I don't want leather edges anyway so I probably wouldn't have had it fixed in any case. I did agree to spend $35 for buttons and loops. Sensible.

Loose notes.

—Every time I get my hair done, the operator says, "What a head of hair!" And each time I cringe. Evil eye. I should have a symbol for it. E squared. Sounds better. (May 30—I was right! They put the wrong color on, four hours of bleaching didn't help, I look ridiculous.)

—I made friends with Mrs. Jacks, the "hostile" woman, at the lab. Not hostile at all. Very talkative, once I began to talk. Also, CBC is "complete blood count." No cancer in it. Hah.

—I meet someone at a performance of *A Doll's House* I haven't seen in twenty-three years. "What's new?" she says, and I look blank. How can I tell her? We talk during one intermission, meet at another, find we're both going to Sarasota next week. Either she or I says something about "surgery," or maybe we don't, but she says she has "to rest." Anyway, it comes out she had a hysterectomy, too. (How in so quick a space of time? How? I know. It's on the tip of her tongue, too. Only she's all right. Do I indicate I'm not? Sort of, I'm sure. Nuts.)

—I can't stop thinking the book is the last one I'm going to write. On the other hand, it may be the last one *you* read (whoever you are).

—Waiting to get into Markham's office, a woman in the hall asks if he's a "good doctor." I tell her he is. "Well," she says, "you shouldn't need him!"

—I read obits. Sixty seems old, until I remember.

—I watch *The Ascent of Man*. Bronowski, dead, but so alive. He says, "All information is imperfect and we have to treat it with humility." On DNA: "Cancer is a gene in the body gone awry." A statement that scares me. I see myself involved in the process of repair and degeneration. Like Darwin's hill—so much is going on; too much for my finite mind to grasp. Watching Bronowski enact Mendel's work with the peas—he talks about ovaries—and I suddenly feel the pain of having had a hysterectomy. (Writing the word now I see it barely registered—too much else superseded it. But I had one, didn't I? And I have a scar. So.)

May 8. Called a friend and found her depressed. Why? Arthur Kober is dying. "He's got cancer. I can't believe it. I don't understand it. I guess we just have to get used to that kind of thing happening." He's at least fifteen years older than I am. I sympathize with her, agree it's terrible.

A few days ago I wrote a condolence letter to my doctor friend Phyllis whose brother died. We had both been at her house soon after our surgery, his for lung cancer. He looked blooming. We compared our good luck. I wrote Phyllis how sad I was. Added I had "confused feelings." Maybe I shouldn't have. But it was true.

The shots and pills seem to be taking hold more than before. It's ten days since my last shot, but I am puffier than ever. My rings barely get on; sometimes I have to use soap to get them off.

Vic has been restless, woke up at five or so this morning and kept waking up. Each time I woke up along with him, and got a numbness in my arm or big toe. Twice I had hot flashes. Is it the added hormone (steroid?), or not having it this week that does it?

I am very flatulent, but then I eat a lot. I am, as Kathy suggested, "being good" to myself. Fat prunes, two candied pears I bought at the spice store, lunch at the Grand Central Oyster Bar. I went to Vic's office, then bought six small clams, a bowl of chowder and a beer (Rolling Rock—at the suggestion of the waiter—straight from Pennsylvania). Who drinks beer in the middle of the day? Me. Am I being neurotically self-indulgent or intelligently self-enhancing? Is it carpe diem or what I should have been doing all along? Would I do it if I thought what I ate (or didn't eat) could keep my weight down? Or if I didn't think taking care of myself was good for me? I even eat cold cereal in the morning. The Geritol lady.

I am going to work on a film strip on health education for Vic. First time in years he's asked me to do anything. What comes to mind? Among other things that I'd better get on with it. Barium enema in June. I would hate to be stopped in midstream. (No pun.) Well, I think, he's been mulling over the project since last October. If I delay it, then I'll have something to pick up at any rate.

I think this journal really ought to end. All it says is that once cancer has been diagnosed, it's always there, like an oil slick in the water, soiling everything.

May 10. For the record—an unpleasant reaction.

My rings have been tight, fingers puffy, general feeling of unease yesterday—and I worked all day in the country preparing for a dinner party and was surprised to find myself very tired by late afternoon. (Was I always? I can't remember. Four months since surgery? Who knows?)

I feel pre-menstrual. Can't figure out whether it is the result of the medication—or the result of it being withdrawn, as my friend Helen feels during her week without Premarin.

At any rate, I went to bed very tired at eleven thirty and woke up at quarter of one, numbness and tingling in my arm and leg (left side this time—the symptoms jump from side to side, fortunately), and feeling faintly nauseated and full in my chest. It feels like water retention, and I shall ask Mark about diuretics. (I just remembered—I woke up in the middle of an erotic dream. In my whole life I can remember only one or two others. It's the fullness.)

I lay quiet for perhaps an hour, a long time actually. Usually I wake up for a minute or two and go back to sleep since what wakes me seems to be (a) Vic's tossing or (b) a physiological something, nothing bothersome in my head. I am very angry (for the first time? I forget so fast). I am angry at Mark for doing this to me (irrational, I know, and even as I catch the thought I am noting it with interest to write down, and I tell myself how crazy it is). I feel *trapped.* There is no escape from the damned thing. The symptoms are so minor, and it is the *treatment,* not cancer, that is annoying me, but it still seems an endless whirlpool. I WANT TO FORGET ABOUT IT. I bedevil myself for not being able to, and at the same time, I realize that if I wake up with a sensation, or can't get my rings off, or have to open my belt, I can hardly be blamed for being reminded.

Barium enema day haunts me too, my father coming up, as he did last time I had tests. The juxtaposition is unnerving.

I must say I write this out of a sense of duty because the truth is that, this morning, I don't feel the way I did in the middle of the night—which I knew would happen at the time.

Now I feel ungrateful and presumptuous.

I AM SO LUCKY. If it is never more than this . . .

And yet the underground stream always murmurs. You get very tired of it. I can see how death can be almost a relief. (The jump from sentence two to sentence three is enormous, but my mind makes it. Again, it is a truth which I must put down, irrational though it may be. I think of Alsop's comment about the constant fear. BUT—he was terminal, wasn't he? And he hurt.)

It's an isolating circumstance. I am myself, whole, living in my world, but inside is this monologue which I have to keep to myself—and mostly do, I think, letting a bit of it surface now and then to Vic and to Helen and to Kathy just in the interest of communication. (I hope I only let a little surface.) Ellen just called and immediately reported on her conversations with Drs. Bernstein and Mark yesterday. She's getting fat and wants to stop the shots (welcome to the club), but no one will let her, although Mark suggests two weeks on and two weeks off. So he can be bargained with! It blows my mind how she intervenes; on the other hand, it's her body. Why not? I yearn to swap symptoms with her —and, despite myself, start—but fortunately she's not interested and cuts me off.

Friend Mark, thank you for this journal. Great prose it ain't, but what a wastebasket!

My symptoms vanish mostly. But I call Mark to check. He says all symptoms are due to medication—and are not permanent but transitory—approves of no salt, mentions diuretics but says we'll try to do without. No sweat.

I am then wiped out until midafternoon.

． ．

May 18. I drive up to the country with Kim and Polly.

Kim, nine, talks of wanting to see the year 2000. She'll be thirty-five. It strikes a chord. I always wanted to see 2000. I would declare, "The millennium has come," a raunchy eighty-five, and presumably expire. I tell Kim it will be wonderful to be around then. She says, "Well, you'll be." I say I don't know. "Oh, sure," she says. But then she starts to talk about death. We are by now driving on Croton Lake Road and the trees are beginning to bud. So we talk about that—each spring reviving the dead winter—the process of renewal—children, in effect, the new leaves and new shoots of their winter grandparents. It's very peaceful and right somehow. (Fantasy—should I write something for them about death and dying? Premature, kiddo, very premature. Forget it.)

To the library. Sneak a look at Kubler-Ross. Always find it a comfort. Why? Her belief in a kind of immortality, I think—"I started not believing anything but the more I work with the dying, the more I am convinced," etc. Also, her picture of the end is not gruesome, it is part of a process. (Am I morbid or trying to find my own philosophy? When I talked to Gottlieb he wanted to know all kinds of specific things about me. All he didn't ask was, "How long are you going to live?" I pointed that out to him and said I could no more answer it for me than I could for him. "Oh," said he, "I'm terrified of dying. I always have been. That's why I can't fly without doping myself up. Every minute of the day I'm scared." Forty-five he is, I think.)

A talk with Kathy.

She had told me earlier that she had gone back into therapy, and I assumed it was because she was now in practice herself. "No," she said, "I've been having problems." She told me some of it—most of it revolving around an Oedipal situation when she was four—and we did have a fruitful talk about it.

Next day, having read the manuscript, she said she hoped I was pushing Gottlieb to do promotion and advertising this time.

"Tell him this time you've no time," she said, or some such thing. There was something about the way she said it that made me say, "It must be a strain for you too, my having been sick," and she got tearful, and then said, "It certainly is. That's really the reason I went back into therapy." "Do you want to talk about it?" If you can take it," she said, and I went over and sat next to her, careful not to put my arms around her. And we talked. Harder for her than for me. Partly because, truthfully, it didn't seem real to me; partly because I could not help being interested in the situation as an observer. At first she said that after the first surgery she was not sure she could go on—"live without you," was her phrase. An astonishing remark, I think. I tried to remember how I felt when my mother had her heart attack, and truthfully I was devastated. But she *was* seventy-three, and I was aware of it, and I must say that each succeeding year, the situation became easier, until at the end, I almost resented her illness, the demands it put on me, and my inability—last spring—to meet them. "Almost" is the wrong word; "resented" is more accurate. I admitted that at twenty-eight, the situation is different. (Even in regard to a child—I remember how important it was for my mother to see Jan, to approve, to "accept the gift.") I told her how hard I was sure it was. But I also said there were pluses. I was well, I intended to continue being well, and yet she was having the experience of facing mortality, valuing life the more, learning something I did not learn (have I?) almost till now.

But then she went on to say that the "worst thing" is that after the second surgery she made her peace with the possibility that I would die, and that she realized she would be able to go on living—and now she felt guilty! I was flabbergasted. The guilt of enjoying yourself when someone you love is in trouble, or ill, or not happy? How well I know that! And how surprised I have been to learn that you are happy when someone you love is happy, all the more if you aren't. At least it has nothing to do with it. Misery does not love company; misery loves the sight of joy. No, she said, it wasn't that. That she knew (that I could rejoice when Helen called in the middle of a difficult weekend to say she and Lewis were having a wonderful time in Vancouver). No, it was just going on with her life if I wasn't around. What she was asking, in effect, was permission. Which I gave.

(What goes on? Is it linked with her four-year-old attachment to me, newly not working, which involved her giving up the care Vic gave her? Is it a revival of an old love-hate?)

Series 4

May 19. Report on the little foxes—swelling, hair, etc. Mark ignores. I don't need diuretics. His ignoring very reassuring somehow. He does tell me of the 200-pound patient before me who is rich but unhappy, never goes to work looking forward to his day, resents being deprived of food and liquor (I don't know the man at all so it's all right to talk about him). I report waking up furious at him, and he smiles.

Later, after I have told him of my fears of being a burden, he tells me of how impressed he is by the way people do carry on under hardship and shares with me his feelings. He speaks of his definition of love: "Being able to break through the barriers, to show yourself to the other person as you see yourself, whether or not it is true. Can you stand this and still love me?" Is that my answer to how much one shares? In part.

Joy of new clothes.

Obituary. Barbara Hepworth, sculptor, dies in fire at seventy-three. Long obituary reports she had cancer of throat. Interviewed at seventy, she said, "You're writing my obituary."

Realize I am so basically hopeful about cures (cure? of

what?) that obituaries puzzle me. How come people die of cancer? How come they're not saved? (When I am able to I don't look to see what people die of.)

Random notes.

Talk with Jan. Mothers of her friends are having "the time of their lives," widowed or divorced. Having affairs. "You'd be great," she says, referring to the past by inference. "I know," I say, and I would be, but I add, "I don't think of myself as a sexual being." A free agent, that is. "I know," she says. "Your mortality." Of course that's what I mean, but it shocks me to have her say it.

We go over old pictures. I tell Kim, "I'm the only one who knows who all these people are." Unsaid—should I mark them? Jan says, "You were so beautiful when you were a child." Same tone in which I look at my mother's baby pictures, same reason I have one framed near my desk. I think how hard it must be for her to live with it. For Vic too. Do I use it? I hope not. Then she says she wants to go to China. Will write embassy in Toronto. "Say you're taking your old parents," I suggest. "They like filial loyalty." "Shall I say you're sick? That'll move them." I'm shocked again. But quickly recover and laugh and say, "By all means."

Driving back to the city there is a new moon. I wish on it. "Life." And am happy to wish it.

Edith buys a Philharmonic ticket series. I say, "I can't," really meaning I don't want to go without Vic. She says, "I know." Shocked again.

Dream. Michael says, "You should live in the country." "Why?" "I'll tell you next year."

(June 1. Dream, again Michael. I am so ambivalent about his joy in Erica and recovery from Sally's death—pleased and threatened for many reasons, I guess. He reports that Sally had found a place in Vermont for him to stay (Erica has a house in East Hampton)—"She saw it last October, she had so much time to look and enjoy herself, she looked wonderful!" Peculiar, but clear. I find it amusing. Sort of.)

. .

May 22. Fifteen pills reduced to ten. (By the week of May 29, when I am typing this, symptoms also seem greatly reduced.)

I walk down a crowded Fifth Avenue at one p.m. to my lunch date at the Plaza (sounds so wonderful!) and look at people rushing around in warm spring day and feel somehow enriched beyond any of them. There is another dimension to my life, no question about it. (In crowded bus I look at people. Am I the only one? I have a secret. Does anyone else? Not scary. Special.)

More stories, books, plays, etc., involving—what else?—cancer. Realize it's the only death a writer can use, other than auto accident or murder. It's both metaphor and extended enough to delineate. Don't get taken in, say I to myself, it's only a device, not an overwhelming fact of life. Okay, kid, deny, deny. (Just realized something. This diary by its very nature is morbid. I shouldn't let *it* fool me either. Or the reader. I should wear a pedometer to check how much time I actually *do* walk through the subject. It can't be as much as it appears here.)

May 26. Day after Memorial Day weekend. A quotation has been running through my mind, or rather, the beginning of one— " 'Hope' is the thing with feathers."

It turns out to be Emily Dickinson (Dickinson and Jane Austen, alone and bursting, how did they sustain it, that infinite internal richness of life?). " 'Hope' is the thing with feathers—/ That perches in the soul—/And sings the tune without the words —/And never stops—at all—"

(I must note that right after that reference in the Bergen Evans dictionary is this one from H. L. Mencken: "Hope is a pathological belief in the occurrence of the impossible." I think the juxtaposition sums it up. Who needs Zen?)

I shall remember that small cheerful bird, because it's true.

As much as the other sings its morbid tune, shrill, piercing, atonic, the little yellow chirp sustains its counterpoint.

It's been an unsettling time, not so much because of anything outside me, as because of my own tight reactions, and what unsettles me is that I don't know whether I am (a) entitled, or (b) should, in the sense that it's healthy, or (c) whether I am becoming a spoiled, demanding woman, like the old mother who is always panting, "My heart!" to get her way.

To wit:

Where shall I start? Maybe Wednesday when I had an hour to kill (fraught word now) between turning over the manuscript, finally, to editor and agent, and meeting Nan at the Plaza for lunch. When I was in the library, looking up the health education material, I found books on hypertension, diabetes, tuberculosis, etc., etc., and sitting next to them a couple on cancer. I did hesitate but if I believe in patient education (I'm not sure I do in this case), I ought to practice what I'm trying to write. So I got the two books too, and got as much—or as little—out of them as the others. It's hard for doctors to cope, chemotherapy is a sometime thing, prognoses are subject to enormous variation (the same tumor that will kill A in six months finds B flourishing after nine years—I, of course, shall be B, at the very least). Came away with a statement that cancer is not "worst of terminal pain." Death is gradual. Anecdote of a woman who says she will "enjoy" the process of dying—and does. Ripeness is all.

At any rate, when I went to the lab on Friday I casually asked Grace, the girl who takes the blood, if there is much variation. She said quickly, "I know, but I'm not going to tell you." I guess she can't—and shouldn't—but it is funny.

I go up to the country then and find the pool filled. I remember when it was emptied in the fall wishing I would live to swim in it again (mixed wish—included in it was the wish that it would belong to someone else by now too). So I go down to swim, saying, "Thank you, God," (God?), en route, and go back and forth for a while. And tell myself going up again, "Be grateful to be able to plan this weekend, be grateful to be of use," etc. And the kids come, and Friday is fine, although I am so sleepy (maybe because I had too much coffee on Thursday, and was up half the night) I go to bed at ten, leaving Vic up, and fall asleep right away.

Saturday I am up early, worried about the planning, about Margit, and the coming of my father next week, and angry at having to be worried about any of it. It is a terribly hot day and I am all swollen. (I cannot get used to the bigness and the puffiness—tough shit, cookie, get used.) But I do a lot, including taking summer things out of closet and putting away winter jackets, and some garden stuff, and realize that I am for the first time in years really *there*—in the house, interested.

And Saturday goes well (Edith and Mollie, another sister-in-law, up). Sunday with Janet's party here is fair—it would have been easier if the weather had been good. The day ends with me absolutely exhausted, so tired I can't sleep again, although on Monday morning I drive into the Bronx, to the hospital and back, feeling great. Why? I am alone. No demands. I wander through Chappaqua trying to find a gas station open and realize I am killing time. I don't want to go back to face—what? Margit? Demands? What for lunch? What is it?

I asked Mark whether medication was making me tired. (When I collapsed Sunday night—after a day of running, true—collapse is the wrong word, anyway; I lay down for a half hour—I said something to Jan about the medication affecting circulation and therefore probably my heart, then hurried to say I wasn't pulling one—was I?) Mark's answer was to show me my counts for the first time—hemoglobin better than last year, before chemotherapy; other count almost like a man's, i.e., I'm not anemic. But he said, "Don't you find you have less tolerance for listening to people or placating them, etc.?" Exactly.

His word is not "tolerance." He said, "Don't you get more impatient?" He also said he does.

(I make a point to tell Vic and Jan about the good blood counts, noting that by making it a point there has been even a consideration of my not, leaving impression medication makes me weak. True? Looks that way, doesn't it?)

I tell Mark about patient education and the lab girl and he laughs, but I seize the opportunity to ask him about my voice. Is it masculinization? I worry about whether I am getting male hormones, well, not worry, am uneasy about it. He says no, it's edema of the vocal chords, and it will not last (presumably after medication stops, first indication that it will stop, if that indeed is what he meant). I also ask if any of the medication is cumulative, i.e., why do I have more symptoms when medication stops for the three weeks? White pills are, he says, that's why the lesser dosage last week. The injected material over the period of five years they've been using it does not accumulate. I do not ask him if the pills or shots affect my sex drive, but I do tell him I have had another erotic dream. (Second in two pill-taking sessions—I'm sure they're linked. Edema of the pelvis? Testosterone? My head? And if testosterone, is it adding something I should have had, or something extra? Who knows? It's not that anything's especially different, just quicker. It's like my friend's mother on Reserpine—she was so much nicer, but we wondered which was the real mother, the one with or the one without? Could just as well have been the Reserpine was filling the lack which had made her such a bitchy woman before.) It was a lovely dream at that. I was going to be raped in a hallway. All the preparations were being made and I couldn't wait. (FINALLY! A RAPE DREAM!) I am escorted to the ghetto-ish scene, and who does the rapist turn out to be? A very polite, smiling, darling, pale-tan Harry Belafonte! Even in my dream, my turning a rapist into H.B. strikes me as so funny that I wake up, alas, before the deed can be consummated.

Back to Mount Kisco and a good time picking spinach and arugala with Jan and all is well until I get boxed in by whether Margit is to drive us back or we are to take the car, whether we are to leave early so Edith can get back and whether Frances and friend can take a sauna and swim (which Vic does not want them to do—that is, he wants no more people in the house, dripping from the sauna, the swimming is okay). But Frances says, "Can I, Vi, please?" and with Vic watching I say yes, and she says I look peculiar, and I say it is because I am fat and puffy. And so we come back into the city and drop everyone off, and Vic says, "Alone at last," and we have a divine time walking on Second Avenue, having a sandwich and beer at some little place, and watching a dopy chase movie on TV. I stay up until midnight (Vic dozing) watching Saigon newsreels. Not tired at all.

And am irritated this morning when bright and early Margit calls to ask funereally, "Are you all right?" "Why shouldn't I be?" "Because you looked strange when you left yesterday." "I'm fine." "But you acted strange. Even Frances asked me." I explain why I looked strange, and even as I write it, my stomach knots.

Damn, damn, damn. I am tired of it. I resent it. I am frightened by it. I have this sense that if only my psyche is okay, I will be, and I resent any threats to it. But—I can't live in a vacuum. Life goes on. It all can't be sweetness and light. Am I entitled to use—I block at the word—okay, cancer, the word cancer—to avoid hassling? When I ask the question, I know the answer. I shouldn't be hassled in the first place, cancer or no cancer. The fact is I don't ask for anything I shouldn't be asking for—the opportunity to live my life as best I can with only unavoidable traumas. I want to work, to do, I don't want to be a parasite, but I don't want to be plucked at!

So! What are you going to do about it? I don't know.

Bob Gottlieb calls to say he's sent the book down to the copy editing department. Finished. "That's a lot of books you've written," he says. "No more amateur." I agree. "Eight," I point out, "including the four novels. And I was a late starter." He says it's a good book and he's pleased to have the dedication, and I say I'm pleased to do it, but I don't ask him if he's going to push this one. Too obvious. I'll tell Lynn. I mention my impatience over the weekend, and he says he's become terribly impatient too. "You've had it with sweetness and light," he says, and I guess I have.

Enough avoiding the film. To work.

May 28. No untoward physical symptoms this series—so far. Even my fingers are less puffy.

Much anxiety though. Why? End of book, difficulty with film script (I finally told myself it isn't my fault I have nothing to write, there *is* nothing to film, Vic is overoptimistic, but there's a reason for the haste—using up the money—and all I can do is the best I can do), boredom (it is excruciating to sit here surrounded by generalities and not be able to write—I realize now how my days this last year have been blessed by something interesting to write—is the latter true? I don't even know how much I wrote or when), and worry about my father's coming. Vic's absence, I suppose. I get stomach pains, the same kind I had last fall when my father came, and I am afraid of the pains. Not so much that they are symptoms as that they may lead to them. Also, I have the barium enema ahead of me. Dilemma: to get it over with, and have the summer—or put it off, and go away to the Vineyard at least, and then come back to it. Last time I got it over with, and couldn't go away (could have too, the surgery proved nothing). Am I assuming they will find something? No, but it's possible. And the possibility divides into two possibilities—it may be important, or, like last time, it may not be. Shit.

Call from Michael. Warm, interested, great. I sounded whining. I was uneasy to begin with, and when he asked how I was, I found it hard to respond in general terms. But to be truthful, over the phone is hard too, because what is my particular truth? It varies all the time. Also, I am very ambivalent about his happiness. Jealous, in a way, because he has so much help in dealing with his own heart anomaly. "I work harder than ever, and I'm not tired." He has his bike, his exercise, Erica, etc. I am jealous of his work, his success in it, his framework, his relationship with Erica. (Also, I feel the connection with Vic—if, when, I die, he'll have the same thing.)

Friday, May 30. I am very angry at myself today because I realize I have been in a mild panic since Gleidman told me I needed a barium enema in the fall and in a real panic since Mark said I should have one in June. The juxtaposition of my father's coming and our plan to go to the Vineyard in July gives me a terrible sense of déjà vu—I walk around convinced something will be found, though not, interestingly, that it will necessarily be any more than was found in January.

I was uneasy all the while Vic was away, except when I saw people, which I realize I should do. It was the being home alone and working, or rather trying to work, that perpetuated the fear. That is, if I am busy, I am not afraid. But the minute I'm not . . .

I realized this when Vic came home last night, a day early. He had called twice the day before to say he would be home Thursday night and I was very pleased. I had wished subliminally on Monday that he would cut it short—for all kinds of reasons— so I came in last night instead of this morning as I had planned. He was at the American Cancer Society meeting and he very casually told me all about it—at length. The statistics, the argument over research and the Cancer Institute programs, and progress in treatment—some good, some bad. I pointed out I had noticed "cancer of the rectum and colon" were among the ones cited as on the positive side. "If detected early," Vic added, and there was a bizarre quality to it all. You would have thought neither of us was concerned at all personally. Then he said he had been asked to head a committee, and I said, "Fine, you can have some influence for me if I need it," meaning I don't know what. (Oh, yes, I do. I will go to NIH or something fascinating and inexpensive—i.e., free—the only problem with that screenplay is what happens to Mark in that case. I have to include him.) Then I tell him the various things I have done or not done, and the people I've spoken to, and I mention casually that I have to have a barium enema, and I'm scared, and should I put it off or get it over with? He blanches. "Get it over with." "No reason," I say quickly, "it's standard," except I haven't mentioned it to him before. "Well," he says, "if you worry, I do." So that's decided. I shall try to set it up even while Dad is here. (Scenario. They find something, but it is so small it can be fixed easily—how easily? Plain surgery? Colostomy? Watch it while chemotherapy takes over? Dr. Ben of nuclear medicine meets me in the hall and says, "I have to level with you." It's December all over again. I think what bothers me is that I thought chemotherapy would be enough, it would be a holding operation, and that's all I would have to think about or cope with. But if that's so, why the careful physicals all the time?) Vic also says, "You have to be watched very carefully for the next five years." Five years? I never think that far. (When Margit asked me if she had a job guaranteed even if we sell the house—she had planned to work another ten years until she will be eligible for social security—I answered yesterday, "I'm really sorry. I don't mean to be morbid, but how can I guarantee you anything? I just don't know. I may live to be eighty—although I doubt it very much—and I may have only a year, who knows? You have to take care of yourself." The fact is I think—and she agrees—that she should go back to Norway where she can be guaranteed health insurance, support if she is ill—which we can't guarantee any more, for reasons that have nothing to do with me. But the truth is that either since the enema was proposed, or I finished the book—both coincided, and I don't know which is the more cogent—I have been in a panic.)

Then we go to bed, and Vic holds me, and after a while he asks if he can put his light back on. He can't sleep. And this morning he is out of bed again at six a.m. and reading in the living room. And I realize—or at least I think I realize—that four days of hearing talk about cancer and talking about it must have been a terrible strain, although he probably doesn't admit it, even to himself. And that's why he came home early. (As a matter of fact, he implied so. So I said I'had felt uneasy with him away, and he said that's why he tried not to stay away any longer than necessary. I said he mustn't let that feeling on my part influence him, but I still feel good that he came back.)

And that is why I am angry at myself again. I keep thinking that I wish the tests were over, and okay, and then—as I said last time—I would "go and sin no more," i.e., try not to think about it.

But, you know, it is almost impossible. Just before I sat down I picked up a book—a rare early morning gesture—to take my mind off this, and page two mentions "A young woman gets cancer, and dies screaming in pain." I CANNOT PICK UP A PAGE OF ANYTHING WITHOUT HAVING MY NOSE RUBBED IN IT. At least so it seems.

But why am I wasting the good time feeling anxious? What can I do about it? Not psychiatry—that I think would be useless. Because what I face is a reality—or is it? What am I afraid of? Even if I should need surgery now—and that is leaping a barrier —I don't think it would be anything final. I would get over it. Until the next time. It's living in limbo that's awful, I guess— can't figure on getting "better," only that nothing gets worse. But what am I saying? That's fine. Would I settle for the status quo? Of course. It's perfectly all right. Except for the fear. (Or is this a plateau I shall climb from too? The end of denial, a facing, and a proceeding from there. Maybe. I shall try to proceed on that assumption.)

May 31. Whether it's the lesser medication or not, I don't know, but all the symptoms have subsided (although my fingers are still puffed).

Kathy comes and reports that Margit told her on the phone that I was to have a barium enema and was worried. (I let it slip when I talked with her about leaving.) I said not really, except neurotically. Then go on to tell her how really good I feel, too, not only physically, but in the sense of life being enhanced, and she smiles strangely. Then says she wrote a story—her first—about our mortality conversation and her feelings about this last year. "It's very heavy," she says. I tell her I'd like to see it, and she says she hoped I would. Permission again. Me with Victor and the novel. I read it and am stunned. For many, many reasons, not least of which is that it is so very well written. She used to be such a Germanic writer—thesis, papers, etc.—this covers some of the ground I tried to in the journal and couldn't, and it is beautiful and moving. Some of it is surprising—the constant telephoning and exchanging of fears between her and Jan, her collapse the first time—although little by little, they've been telling me about it. Parts about Vic are very moving. And she has our conversations down pat. But what is unnerving—and it *is* unnerving—is to be done to as I have done, to be made a character. She said at the start, "Don't think I know anything you don't, because I don't." Why? She writes of me as if I were dead. As a matter of fact, the story says, "My mother is dying." It goes on to tell how my behavior this last year has changed her, freed her, inspired her, etc., and ends (if I remember correctly—she is sending me a copy, and should, because like the patient listening to a doctor after the shock of diagnosis, I really don't remember it very well) on a very upbeat note. But I am also a little angry (I am being buried) and a little scared (evil eye business) as well as set up (all I have to do is be noble, and I will not be a burden but a privilege, hah!) and put out about the good writing (a compliment to her—no mother preening over a child, a colleague being jealous of another) and disturbed at my disguise being broken (if it is published, as it should be, may well be) and amused (how many disguises do *I* break!). But I understand and am really unequivocally pleased that she has discovered the secret—that by making fact into fiction you free yourself (as indeed she has—she wrote the story and told her psychiatrist she was finished, except to show it to me and send it to him—he is a character in it too). And she has done something for me as well that is very, very important. By making me into fiction for herself, she has made that part of me into fiction for *myself,* and I have not been scared or morbid since! (It may not last, of course, but some of it will stick.)

June 1. The Collins wedding. Hassidic guests, members of the bride's family, giving a whole new dimension with their dancing and prayers. A really moving and exciting business.

Afterward, the sun appearing briefly, I strike up a conversation with one of the bride's mother's friends and we go for a walk in the woods. We come upon her husband talking and she mutters, "The camp, always he talks about camp." At first I think she means summer camp, but fortunately I realize quickly and ask her if she was in "the camps." She says, "Yes, and so was he." And we talk about it, and she says it is always present, the memory, an underground river, and she cannot escape because she feels so guilty at having survived. Not new to me, of course, but I have never heard anyone say it, least of all a handsome, well-dressed woman walking in a Bedford wildlife garden. We talk about it earnestly, and I ask her if life isn't enhanced at the same time. Doesn't she feel more conscious of knowing what is important and what isn't? Didn't she, I ask urgently, get any good out of it? (Isn't there some good to be gotten out of the Holocaust? asks Pollyanna.) But she won't buy. "No," she says firmly, "no, seeing your mother and father and sisters and brothers die, no, nothing. I am guilty." "But think how terrible it would be for all of us if none of you survived? How important it is for all of us?" This holds her for a moment. Then she shakes her head. How can I understand? But I do, and I say what is underneath all of my talk, of course. "I have gone through something of my own," I say. "Cancer. I'm fine," I add hastily, and she says, "Thank God," and I go on, "But life is in some ways richer because of it, it isn't all blackness." I plead with her to make the concession. And you know what? We kept on talking, but I can't remember what she said then.

·   ·

Evening. Mrs. Markham has called, Margit says. "Call the hospital to make other arrangements."

A pall.

"Shall I call for you?" says Vic.

I shake my head. Call Mrs. Markham at home. A cold with fever. Good. "Give him my love."

How dependent I am. What a burden we must be for him! He's our lifeline.

Permission for Mark. Of course we would survive. Promise. But it would be hard.

I write Sissman a rambling, presumptuous, bumbling, but genuine letter about his poem. I've been meaning to for months, but something makes me do so today, so I do.

I keep thinking I should do something about Transcendental Meditation. Learn it as someone about to be blind learns Braille. As a prop. (Mother's words—everything, Christian Science especially, a prop.)

Some of my anger at myself last week was a realization that in worrying I do what I was so angry at Mother for doing. Wasting the perfectly good present in fear about the future. I read somewhere—worry is fantasy, it's imagining what may not ever be. Mine is a little realistic, though. But wasn't hers? She did have a coronary, she did live with angina. He jests at scars, right, Mother. A year tomorrow that she died.

If I were to have a mantra, it should be the word "Control." That's what all my worry is. An effort to anticipate in order to be able to control. Blessed are the uses of uncertainty. Great are the joys of being out of control. (Even writing the last is frightening. I had a sense of going down a roller coaster.)

From *The Lives of a Cell:* " 'The long habit of living,' said Thomas Browne, 'indisposeth us to dying.' "

"Perhaps we would not be so anxious to prolong life if we did not detest so much the sickness of withdrawal."

"We may be about to rediscover that dying is not such a bad thing to do after all. Sir William Osler took this view: he disapproved of people who spoke of the agony of death, maintaining there was no such thing."

"I have seen agony in death only once. . . ."

"I find myself surprised by the thought that dying is an all-right thing to do, but perhaps it should not surprise. It is, after all, the most ancient and fundamental of biologic functions, with its mechanisms worked out with the same attention to detail, the same provision for the advantage of the organism, the same abundance of genetic information for guidance through the stages, that we have long since become accustomed to finding in all the crucial acts of living."

On Death in the Open: "It does make the process of dying seem more exceptional than it really is, and harder to engage in at the times when we must ourselves engage."

"There are 3 billion of us on the earth, and all 3 billion must be dead, on a schedule, within this lifetime. The vast mortality, involving something over 50 million of us each year, takes place in relative secrecy."

"We will have to give up the notion that death is catastrophe, or detestable, or avoidable, or even strange. We will need to learn more about the cycling of life in the rest of the system, and about our connection to the process. Everything that comes alive seems to be in trade for something that dies, cell for cell. There might be some comfort in the recognition of synchrony, in the information that we all go down together in the best of company."

Coming out of the movie *Hearts and Minds,* I think what kind of world is this that I should wish to live on in it.

All I want is not to be a burden to Vic. My heart palpitates and I feel it with joy. Maybe that is what I will get—death suddenly—but not for a while. There is too much to live for right now.

. . .

Allan Greg on dying in the *Difficult Art of Giving:* "The big payoff of this last stroke has been . . . a substantial change of my old-time aversion to death; it's not a vivid thing at all—just a slow and rather dull and partial bit of stupidity, and drowsiness. It's a charmingly different set of values and motivations from what I had ever experienced or imagined . . . I've been right near it, and realize that you have to be pretty much alive to fear anything. So I feel heartened and adjusted, in a fresh and cheerful mood."

From an interview with Beverly Sills, post-cancer, pre-Met debut: "One thing my surgery taught me; don't make too many plans."

"I'm a complete cure," says she. Good for her.

"A life so wildly unbalanced, traced with the sunniest hills and the most terrifying values." Visits to her retarded, epileptic son so "emotionally pulverizing, the one defense is a constant cheerful smile."

Who could honestly be astonished that on the eve of her Met debut, the only house she hadn't sung at, they'd tell her she had cancer?" The evil eye again.

"Perhaps it's because I'm too young, or perhaps because I can't be afraid, death does not terrify me in the least. I'm affected only because other people are saddened by it and because I myself would miss that person, but otherwise nothing. It happens; perhaps you live somewhere else, and that is nothing to be afraid of; perhaps you just sleep. Those you leave behind miss you but in the long run all of us work out our own salvation. I would not be afraid to die and I should want no sorrow or fuss for me." From a letter by Violet Brown (to be Weingarten) to her mother at the age of seventeen or so!

June 3. The last of Series 4. Mark, wan, with mask, cheerful and helpful. Asks me how I am. I tell him, truthfully, fine. No treatment symptoms (since fewer pills). So far, since Kathy's story, no fear. I say I know Vic called him, but I tell him the context in which I mentioned the barium enema. "It's only a test," he says quickly, and I point out that I know this, only I am "neurotic."

Which word he seizes upon. "Nobody likes to have an enema," he points out, "and if there is a possibility of bad news in it, it is realistic to worry. Why do you demean yourself by saying you are neurotic?"

I explain. He asks by way of reply whether I know anyone who doesn't worry, even about so minor a thing as a Pap smear. I say yes. Michael, with his heart. Anne with a once cancerous kidney, now removed, "to which I never give a thought." "Do I believe that?" I admit that I do.

So we talk, wonderfully, about how different people take vicissitudes, about our fear of not measuring up, of how, really, our past determines our present actions. I go through my litany of the positives in all of this—and he insists that if the sky is bluer for me now (when it is blue), it always must have been, or at least I must have been able to see it. What he is trying to say is "trust yourself." And I hear it. And as usual I walk out feeling equipped to handle—what? Life. For, of course, as we point out, we are talking about life and health, not death and sickness. He also says we will put off the famous barium enema. (I have suggested we have it at once.) I protest, but with a nod to the evil eye in the corner, I agree. It *is* a good idea. Why should not weakness (is that the word?) be acknowledged and accepted too? Caliban—this thing of darkness is my own. Or is it strength—yes, this is how I am, today, this month—so be it.

I am a little uneasy about the preceding pages I gave Mark. So raw. So unedited. So unwritten. But that's how the truth appears. So be it again.

Yesterday was the anniversary of my mother's death. Not today. I, who never even to this day forget my grandmother's birthday, got the day mixed up. Why? Because I am so insistent on my own mortality? Strange.

Back Trouble

June 6. Wonders continue. I go to meet my father, nervous as usual. Wait at the gate (having gotten through security by saying he is "an old man, he'll be nervous if he doesn't see me"), and at 11:30 the grandparents start coming out the door. Elderly, halting, gray, nervous. At the end of the line a blooming, smiling man in an elegant new blue shirt, new pants, new shoes. Who? My "old" father. En route to the baggage claim he confides he was driven to the airport in Fort Lauderdale in a "brand-new Bentley." Whose? His new "friend's." Zsa Zsa Gabor type, she sounds. About "fifty-nine, but she looks younger." He is reborn. No more shuffle. No more tears. She bosses him. Made him buy new clothes. Scolds about his shabby apartment. I go to get the car, delighted and a bit shaken too, because already he has told me she has described my mother as "she was an old woman, she wasn't interested, but you . . ." Hah! I powder my nose and comb my hair before I start the car.

Later he tells me more. Says one must live from day to day. I have fantasized a few wise heart-to-heart talks, right? Mostly about me, I guess. Sharing over the generations! Hah, again. A day later he has still asked me nothing about me. Only talked about himself. He sounds and acts half his age. (Half his? Half mine!) He does say he "feels guilty" even though he knows he is free. I tell him I understand, and assure him he shouldn't feel guilty at all. (Who, me? Ambivalent?)

Through the looking-glass!

Life is truly irresistible.

June 7. 7:30 a.m. I want to write it before I talk it, because while it's not irrational, I sense it's no one's fault. It's a phenome-

non which I shall have to deal with. Interesting. May be helpful
to be facing, because it is certainly there—the underground
stream. (Is the fear the mask for it? If depression is a mask for
anger suppressed, fear may be too.)

Yesterday's entry was true—as was Kathy's story, which she
just sent and which we reread. But only *a* truth. In many ways,
both represent a cover, and a denial. The saint of Kathy's story is
mostly whistling in the dark. And I didn't, until one o'clock this
morning, have any notion of what she meant by asking permission
for life to go on. Not the slightest. Now I do. Not in terms of
her—that still remains emotionally clear—but certainly in the
following.

It started last night when we we all went to the fair and I
gave Vic what he perceived as the wrong directions. (Actually not,
but that's irrelevant.) And he blew up at me—in front of Jan,
Kim, but most important of course, my father. And instead of being apologetic I was outraged. I didn't hide it, for once, either from
myself, or from him (Jan's anger was a buttress). He did apolo-
gize, and later, at my behest, pointed out that being given directions in a car, which put him in a dangerous (to him) position,
angers him unreasonably. True. But for me it was—click! Why
wasn't his first impulse—thinking I was wrong—to reassure me,
as I would have him? Or to cover up his anger because I would be
embarrassed in front of my father? Or not to—vital—scold poor
little vulnerable me! Considering. (Later I thought it was a compliment, wasn't it? He isn't self-conscious about poor me. At one
a.m.—before I got up and took a Valium. Sensible? Admission of
failure to cope?)

Anyway my anger grew. And I was angry that all my life was
spent being afraid of—*is* spent being afraid of—and wanting to
please my father and my husband, who are going to have a wonderful time when I am gone, which I will be soon. (I know, it's
Oedipally mixed. But pleased, delighted, relieved though I am at
Dad's new interest—and a bit worried too, because Zsa Zsa may
very well hurt him—I also remember that she said my mother's

house was a disgrace because she was an "old woman," and I see him buying new clothes, going to good restaurants, while my mother—my mother had to fight to get her television fixed! Later I realize it was her fault too, in a way—she should have spent what she had, or insisted. But she did insist. She tried. And in the end she just didn't care, I guess.) Back to Kathy's wanting permission for life to go on. I am angry for the first time at not having made the most of things when I could have. It translates materially too—although that's only a symbol. I fantasized leaving Vic, divorcing him (provoking him into giving me reason by not waiting around all the time for him to come back and leaving him alone—old fear emerging—which he knows because he is meticulous about letting me know where he is and where he will be), running. Where? Away. At times like this, my world is like an old map—all the edges point out that there are demons as soon as one reaches the limits. I spend my life waiting—waiting for the car, or to drive someone, or for doctors' appointments, or for Vic to come home. I am always at the edges of what appear to be other people's active lives—waiting, reacting, never my own center. That's always been true, and even as I write, I realize it's my own choice, and desire. My life is here, at the typewriter; not my whole life, but my working life. Not in Louisville, or Maine, or even going to an office.

Anyway. On my own I realize I have nothing material that is my own. Nothing. Even the car, I gave away. And that is wrong. But I did it, with my eyes-closed-to-anything-I-accomplished attitude. And all the time that I am thinking—angrily—I am writing the figure 40 on my left hand with my right. Later it becomes 40,000, and I become interested enough to stop to figure out what it means.

I can't.

But this morning I wake up at seven and I realize 40 is a figure meaning the limitless. Well, it's like this. The Hebrews said it rained forty days and forty nights, i.e., a long time. Like Methuselah living nine hundred years. Also a symbolic figure. I am so pleased with my subconscious dredging that up in the middle of my anger that my anger evaporates. One of life's fascinations.

I am, of course, not angry now. At least the reality has left me. (So has the backache and stomach ache I had yesterday.) But I have a sense that this is important. To face the anger, admit it. It isn't a desire for anyone to be unhappy. I don't think so. It would be illogical certainly. But a fact—the ambivalence Kathy caught —is anger that someone else (and I guess who) will unleash the kind of joy and new life I see in them all—Michael, my father (Vic?). Would I not feel it if we were less boxed in now? That's certainly a part of it. But I also realize that in this I am literally a spoiled brat. Sitting at my typewriter in the country with a maid fixing breakfast (and what of the woman who has to worry about who will take care of her child? or pay the bills? or run the house when she dies? I complain because I can't go to Paris and stay at the Ritz. Harsh? A symbol? Sure, but you pick your symbols, don't you? Maybe it's a metaphor. If I am going to face the anger, I can't scold myself for its unacceptable manifestations. Lack of nobility.).

It would really be interesting if I am angry, not afraid. Or a little of both. There is no single truth, only many truths. I somehow respect the anger more at the moment.

I think that the happiest time of my mother's life came when she was over sixty and they did their traveling. I don't want to be cut off or cut back. I don't want to feel like a temporary interim block in what is going to be a good life for Vic. My nose—oh, how marvelous—is out of joint because my father has a girl younger than me (she says).

I want to cry.

Poor me. Not poor little me. Poor me. Poor all of us humans who have to endure life as best we can and put up our puny defenses to do so and can't kid ourselves all the time about how puny they are.

Although—again, here, truthfully—my defenses don't seem so puny.

On chemotherapy, I feel fine. None of last time's untoward reactions.

I guess I won't run away.

Forty. Very interesting. (The things I want? The indefinite time I wish I had? Do have. Defenses up.)

June 24. The day of the bone scan. The trouble with a journal is that you have to write it every day because everything changes. Unfortunately I couldn't write the last two weeks.

Monday after the last Saturday's entry I literally could not move. Lower back pain. Standard. Ashamed because Vic has lived with it so long and gone about his business so uncomplainingly. Right away the thought—how can I stand pain? How will I be? (No connection with possible tumor—well, not very much connection—but logically, if Mark and Dr. Haberman, the orthopedist, want a bone scan there must be a possibility. I hope not. Anyway.)

Vic called Mark and Mark insisted that I come up, and I did—really in agony. He found little, I think, and sent me to Dr. Haberman, who seemed to me to find little too—long notes dictated in my presence indicated nothing. Yesterday, however, Mark mentioned a "small nodule"—first I say whatever that is, now I pause to look it up. Sorry I looked it up—"small rounded mass or lump." Situation begins to change, but I shall try to keep the feeling of the past weeks anyway. I did have X-rays. Presumably they were clear. I was told to rest, take Valium, Percodan. Really enjoyed—in a way—the next period. I went to Boston for Kathy's graduation—by plane, instead of car—and maybe because of medication, liquor, etc., really felt little or no pain. Friday went to cemetery with Dad, kids, and Jan—saw Mother's tombstone, made no impression. Like her funeral.

Still, all the while I had a sense of peace (Valium?), as if my soul was catching up. I read, rested. My father managed to keep himself busy at track, ballet, walking, and all in all, we had the most relaxed time we had ever had together.

The pain seemed to diminish but not so much. Last weekend, cutting down on medication, it seemed as bad as it had two weeks ago. But I felt stronger, more agile.

Read a quote from Henry James—"So here it is at last, the distinguished thing," meaning death. Took him three months after that. Copied it down, but I had no feeling. I really have not thought once about cancer during the last two weeks. Only about my ability to bear pain without mentioning it. Realize it isn't very great. And I guess nothing else matters at that point—you either hurt, or you don't. Philosophy, behavior, manners, irrelevant. Too bad.

On Sunday I lie flat under the sky for a while. Remember how I watched an eclipse of the sun in the pool and how lovely it was. Feel very peaceful. Maybe we shouldn't sell the house. I should just lie here under the trees. (No reality in the thought . . . note that description of "'nodule" is making me commit typos.) I think I've had it all really—like Darwin having evolution on the hill slope outside his window. I haven't ventured far, but I do think I've experienced a lot. Except old age. When I told Kathy I had a bad back, she exclaimed, "Why are you getting so old all of a sudden?" So maybe I'm having that, too.

I think how sympathetic Vic is (but pain is a separating device—you really think only of yourself). I think—this is Sunday, under the trees—I think of this pain as a kind of preview, a foreknowledge—and remember how I memorized poems to say to myself while I was in labor with Jan. Hah! You can't prepare yourself for pain. You are simply trapped until it untraps you. (As I am now. Haberman gave me an injection which until this moment —11:30 a.m. the next day—has really made me comfortable.)

Monday, I find I can sit in the chair to have the temporary filling put in last January made permanent. I manage an hour and a quarter, pain-free (which is more than this typewriter bit is). Novocain? Good thoughts? Who knows? I try it on myself waiting for Mark yesterday—really in pain after an hour of waiting in the house and driving myself up—and for a few minutes after I see him I can't locate any pain. Fortunately the spell goes.

Also got a call from Kathy saying a "Mr. Weingarten" has been trying desperately to reach her and she has been desperately calling Vic who has gone to Maine. (He spoke to Mark before he went, knew about the scan, says "he tells me the truth," didn't sound scared, would he have gone if . . . ? But that was before the "nodule" remark. Knock it off.) I get torn about telling her that I am having the scan—if Vic tells her and I don't she gets sore, on the other hand . . . I tell her casually after she has told me she solved the "Mr. Weingarten" calls. She has a new secretary —at least the office has—and when Hilary, her husband, called and told her to "call her husband," the girl kept writing "Weingarten" instead of "Worthen." So I didn't have to tell her. Shouldn't have.

May I please learn to keep my mouth shut, never mind they say I should level with them.

I hope it's nothing. I hope I don't need radiation. Doesn't chemotherapy—or rather isn't chemotherapy supposed to take care of such?

Until the next chapter.

P.S. I wish I would stop fashioning scripts. Here I get the barium enema postponed and I'm back to tests anyway. I feel very sorry for Mark. I keep feeling I fail him every time I'm not blooming.

June 25. So far as a preliminary reading can tell, the scan is okay. I met Dr. Haberman in the tunnel to Van Cortlandt (feeling cheerful—oddly, as soon as I get to the hospital, its own remote world sets in) and mentioned the word "nodule." Said I had heard it, but I had just dared to look it up. "Fifty percent of patients have 'em," he said. "Trouble with dictating in front of patients." He grinned, I patted his cheek. Made lying with the moving finger writing somewhat easier.

This morning, though, seems a kind of end of innocence. Dr. ?, who looked at the scans briefly, said they seemed okay but "check with Dr. Markham tomorrow afternoon when we've gone over them more carefully." They looked red—liver scan was "perfect" when it was white—obviously what I do not know about nuclear medicine is considerable. Anyway normally I would be euphoric—or, at least, totally reassured. Not now. I felt well enough to take the bus down, since it appeared on the street when I did, and even a second bus home since it was pouring, but no sense of "now I'm free again." First, I want Mark to tell me. Second, it is only reprieve. Third, the injection is wearing off (now, this morning) and my back hurts. I know. I shouldn't be sitting at the typewriter, but what difference does it make really? With a bad back you go on until it stops.

The end of innocence is something else. Monday I reminded Mark he had forgotten to give me the prescription for my "cancer" pills. He laughed and corrected. "Alkeran." Okay, it does say that on the bottle. I barely looked before. He had said to Vic on the phone that if I were a "healthy young person" he would say the back has two to four weeks to go and forget it, but under the circumstances . . . Well, I feel like a "healthy young person." Or did until now. Now—at this moment—everything I write, think, or feel, I realize, is "at this moment." I feel like an alcoholic who has finally admitted it. (I have a faint recollection of having made the same comment a while back, but that is a point, too. All, as someone once remarked, is flux.)

I got back to the apartment and the elevator man was aghast at the plane crash that had just occurred at Kennedy. I watched on television—interested, but not aghast. All I could think was, "It was quick." In terms of the passengers. Not the survivors. I also thought of Vic coming in tomorrow; Jan, today. *That's* different.

Stayed with Judith for a while during the interim between the nuclear draft (how we take such things for granted—one man next to me, a black, was going to the beach in the interim—true, he arrived too late afterward to get the test, as it turned out, so maybe there is such a thing as being too casual—or too afraid . . .). She was so pleased with how she is making do with only one maid—the cook on vacation—sounds funny, but it really isn't. She takes pulses, blood pressures, makes the sandwiches, etc. But what she really was saying was how pleased she is to be able to take care of her husband. I said it was different with a woman. "Stephen could never do it," she said. "He even goes to the diner for breakfast if he is alone in East Hampton." "No," I said, "I don't mean that. I mean a woman is used to taking care— she feels enhanced—but when she has to be taken care of . . ." "You're right," she said. And it *is* different. I feel sad and a little guilty that I can't do the film for Vic. And it is painful, but need-ful, for me to be typing, but I understand that the macho factor is missing too. I am *not* failing to take care of my empire, or earn my living, or being tough. On the other hand, I am not the amiable —what? Housewife? That's denigrating. Again, in my head as well as in my back, this has a different connotation. As it should. It does for Mark and Haberman.

Back to "I am a cancer patient." Does it change things? I'll have to see. Maybe it will be a relief. Instead of Rebecca of Sunny-brook Farm inside, a grownup, trying to decide when to say "can-cer" pill and when to say "Alkeran." (I can never spell the name of medications. But the answer is fairly evident. Don't mention it, if you can avoid it. Use the right name, casually, if you must. Hon-esty is a touchy business here. You have to gauge how much di-rectness makes people more comfortable—and how much doesn't. The word has lost some of its terrors for me—I think—but I guess it hasn't for others.)

To bed—and how wonderful that was, after a beer and a sandwich and two Tylenols, or maybe a Percodan. (I take Perco-dan like forbidden fruit. Why?) I remember Louise Dooneiff say-ing that one of the pleasures of being ill was being able to rest. Alas.

Then, catching up with the *Times Book Review,* I came upon
Kathryn Ryan's piece about Connie. It begins, "Cornelius Ryan
died on Nov. 23, 1974, in Memorial Sloan-Kettering Hospital in
New York City. His last book, *A Bridge Too Far,* was No. 2 on the
best-seller list. He had begun work on a fourth book about World
War II and its outline is scrawled in one of two notebooks he kept
at his bedside table."

The other notebook was this one, apparently. Since 1970, it
said, when his cancer was first discovered, he had made research
trips to five countries, interviewed over two hundred specialists in
radiology, chemotherapy, research, and surgery, and talked to more
than five hundred cancer victims. He interviewed nurses, doctors,
technicians and, at the end, patients in the hospital. The journals,
say Kathryn, "reveal the intellectual arguments he conducted with
himself on how best to face the inevitability of a death for which no
date is set and no pardon is foreseen." Beautifully put. That last is
what it is all about.

And how fascinating! Again—I think—man versus woman.
Certainly monumental Irish ego versus—okay, me.

The Erbanses had been telling me about his battle (long before it became pertinent to me). The trips, the French Legion of
Honor, the entrees to famous doctors, the refusal of medication
so he could type his manuscript, the sweat of pain running down
his face. No money (possible, that?), but a huge household, sec-
retaries, Kathryn researching, everything revolving around HIM—
his pain, his cure, his work—and, I would assume, no guilt on his
part, far from it, he was writing to take care of them all. He was
writing a best-seller and lived to see it so (and be visited by Prince
Bernhardt at the end).

The Christmas before the last, he had a great ball—musicians,
dancing, black tie, flowers, all the famous. He ordered a giant gay
wake. (Did he have it? I doubt it. No one told me.)

He also said that he was not writing about generals, but
about "kings," ordinary men who were able to find the courage

they needed in battle. He was writing about himself—a "king " who was looking for the courage he needed.

But five hundred interviews! Five countries! Two hundred specialists! Keep moving, and let everyone move with you.

I keep looking for the "king" too—okay, "queen"—inside me. My journeys take place on the head of a pin. Microcosm versus macrocosm. All the same, I think. He did do it very well. The Gordons said they never admired him—or her—more. What a way to go! (Hah—another phrase that comes alive!)

All I can think of at this point—wryly, my back hurts too much for me to go on (no Ryan tears rolling down my cheeks for me—not for this)—is that maybe old Gottlieb will put an extra ad in the *Times* for me. Because of. But do you want to know something? I don't want to be advertised, admired, loved, etc.—"because." I am a "healthy young woman" of sixty (oh, dear, I am a nut!) with a bad back—I hope. Am I going to wait for Mark to call me or am I going to call him?

What would Ryan have done? Commandeered a helicopter and sent a platoon to the Bronx to bring back doctor and scans to be explained to him in person!

I should have been born Irish.

Two hours later.

I decide I am Irish enough to call. Mark busy on phone. Jane, his secretary, says he will call back.

An hour later.

Jan is back from Dallas—unexpectedly—and wants to come over for a sandwich. Since I expected her to be Mark, I sounded scared and had to tell her why. (Had to? Did. So be it.) Also asked her not to come over but promised to call as soon as he did. I think I am better suffering alone. And I am suffering. Not only in my back—unimportant, that—but I am terrified. Why? Why is

this day different from all others? Because the longer it takes me to
hear, the more I think they are discussing what to do about me—
and I do not want to tell Jan or Vic or Kathy. I am also afraid of
pain. Pain makes you helpless. Selfish. I am in a true panic. Why?
Why? Why? I lie like a stone until after four when Mark calls to
say that all has been checked and is negative, rest, and he will see
me Monday. Reprieve.

This morning I read about the plane victims and weep—not
for the dead ones, for the burned suffering ones. Why don't they
let them slip away? Why let a little girl of seven survive burned
from head to toe? Who am I to decide?

If I got into such a panic, I clearly have made peace with
nothing. What was this all about? I obviously hurt before—but I
don't remember. I hurt now—but it has no emotional significance.
So are there two kinds of pains? Ones that will end, and ones that
will not? Was pain what made this one different?

I remember thinking—with awe and joy—in the midst of
unmedicated labor with Jan (wartime, I didn't yell, so they let me
alone all night) that every being ever born came this way.

Everyone who ever dies must go through the same process
too. My God, it's not a matter of jesting at scars—you simply cannot understand. But what is there to understand? That it is unpleasant, nagging, sometimes painful—is that helpful? I really
don't know what I feel right now—except like a healthy young
woman of sixty with a backache!

Maybe that's what's interesting—the mystery. But then I
sound like an American woman delegate at the International
Women's Conference in Mexico. The Third World people talk
about the woman of Zaire rising at dawn, baby on her back, to chop
cane for ten hours, walk three miles for water, cook dinner, and
then start all over again after a few hours of rest (and impregna-
tion?). *Our* delegates talk about women getting the same amount
of federal money for football at college as the men—not that bad
usually but that indeed is what was on the morning news!

Well, you are what you are. The lady from Zaire doesn't lie

like a stone waiting for a telephone to ring (or is that only a different version of Orientals having no regard for human life—"kill their babies, means nothing to them, bud"!). I don't know.

I am what I am.

(Even that is a bit Godlike. Isn't that what He says somewhere in the Old Testament? I AM THAT AM. Maybe that's the ultimate truth. What is, is. Period! Have I learned anything from this episode? I don't think so. Or is that in itself learning something?)

July 20. Nearly a month since the last entry, and as I force myself to sit down, I am again conscious of great anger. I don't *want* to write anything—at least, not in this journal. Why? (As I write the foregoing, even the process of writing down my unwillingness eases the anger. It is as if I am forcing myself into a process, and despite myself, I feel the beginning of enjoyment at being involved. I have been like the Ancient Mariner stranded on that painted ship upon a painted ocean. Barren. Shipwrecked on a raft. A month! A blank month! My God!)

Somewhere amid the papers on my desk I find an old scrawl from *On Aggression* by Konrad Lorenz—"A personal bond, an individual friendship, is found only in animals with highly developed inter-specific aggression . . . Biologically, love is only possible where there is anger—and hate." He also says (and I just write it down because I like it—it has nothing to do with the process I am trying to start here): "The long-sought missing link between animals and the really humane being is ourselves."

Maybe acceptance is possible only where there is anger and hate, and this is a month during which I have allowed both to flourish inside me. About being incapacitated, I mean. Strong word, but that's what it feels like. I resent it. But I don't feel I have to keep it to myself. A bad back is an ailment it is possible to talk about. It is permissible to bitch about it. *Everyone* has it. *Young* people have it. (First time I turned up with it, Mark told me his son had been caught with so bad a spasm he had to be taken to the hospital for an injection before he could move.)

Let me see if I can recapitulate what has happened inside me. (I haven't been able to sit at the typewriter long enough to write before now. It still hurts, but in a qualitatively different way. And I can't write except at a typewriter. My thoughts go out through my fingers.)

My last entry was cynical. I thought the tests were over, but even so, I wasn't particularly happy. Something else would happen. It always does.

And it did. The following Monday Mark said he wanted an IVP. Okay. I was still pain-free enough to ride around the countryside to meet Marian Erbans for lunch (a kind of Last Lunch?), and went through the castor oil, and had the test—and again, was scared. "It looks okay," said the doctor, "but check with Dr. Markham tomorrow." Repeat of previous week's day of anxiety. All clear.

Why do I get so scared?

Why have I not adjusted to the fact that what will be will be? (*Times* obit of Ozzie Nelson—dead of liver cancer—"He took the situation with great equanimity and died serenely"—words to that effect anyway. Or did he? Is it maybe another chapter of *Ozzie and Harriet?* Immaterial, either way.)

The next Monday—last of Series what? 5?—Mark says he would like me to see a neurologist. Just to make sure it isn't a disc. (It is though. Probably. Bill Collins said so last October after taking X-rays. Apparently he didn't communicate same to Mark. I thought he had.) And for the first time in all of this doctoring I go on strike inside. I make the appointment all right—but for three weeks hence, the same day I am to come back to see Mark for Series 6. I make it clear to the secretary in neurology that it's no emergency, and so she gives me the last date. "Weren't you here before?" she asks. And of course I was. To see Dr. Weitzman. Enough of doctors! I take charge of myself for the first time. I decide I will give myself a solid week of rest (interrupted, true, by going out to dinner a couple of times), or maybe two. And then I will be better.

And I do just that. Rest. Read. Some days I go out not at all. And I think I am better. I hurt, true. (Physical recap for the record—sort of a chronic mild backache, occasionally going down right leg, but not into big toe, especially in the morning, and also occasionally veering into right hip, at which time back does not hurt, or into lower abdomen, at which time back continues to hurt. Pain at the moment may be ascribed to two causes—twelve hours upright yesterday because of lunch company who stayed until after six and then a dinner engagement—or swimming both yesterday and today, the pool having reached a temperature of 80 degrees. I called Dr. Haberman on Friday—out of a sense of duty to myself —and said, "How long, oh Lord?" and he said, "A day, or infinity." What more? Aspirin is better than Tylenol to ease the inflammation in the back, and I should do what I can do. Use my own judgment. Swimming is a calculated risk. It may not help the back but it helps arms and wrists. A note on that—wrists have been aching since I took to my back—no Freudian slip, that, that's exactly what I've done. Why? Maybe because they're used to being used typing and are sore for lack of exercise. Or maybe because they're part of the circulatory problem I had during the spring post-chemotherapy.

Of the chemotherapy, except possibly the wrist phenomenon and the damned fuzz on my cheeks, no bad signs. I have even lost weight—six pounds maybe. I still can't wear my wedding ring or diamond, but the edema is so lessened I can get into the size 10's again. I am still over 120 pounds, so I have only the slightest, most infinitesimal wonder whether the weight loss is (a) significant in a bad sense or (b) is a sign that the chemotherapy isn't as effective. On the other hand, my voice gets lower and lower. Met new people yesterday who commented on how "husky and velvety" my voice is. My voice! Betty Boop, whispery teenaged

voice that came over the radio the time Arlene Francis taped me. I
listen to it. It's different. No question. I can't shout either, but then
I never could. Mostly I think none of us hears the difference.

July 21. Got started on this yesterday, but Vic came home
early. End of journal.

This morning started with the *Today* show. A Mrs. Leibman
in bed at Mount Sinai, totally paralyzed by myasthenia gravis. A
wire coming from her ear, so I assume she hears the interview
with her doctor. She is the "worst" case they have. Later we are to
see their "best"—a young girl probably cured, a young woman
still under treatment but resentfully, I think, from the expression
on her face, said to be on her way. Why put Mrs. Leibman
through that horror? Why did I look? There but for the grace of
God? There, by the grace of God, soon? Who knows? I suppose
Mrs. L. thought allowing herself to be shown was a way of serving.
Like this journal, I suppose. Poor Mrs. L. I'd like to write her, but
anything I can think of saying would sound patronizing. No
answer, incidentally, to my letter to Sissman. I shouldn't have done
it, I guess. Still it was no invasion of privacy. He wrote about it. If
Kathy's story appears—and Anne says it is very good—I have
asked her to do it under her "married," not her "birth" name—a
request she takes pretty hard. "What irony!" she said. "You
wanted to write under your own name and felt you should do it
under your married name, and it's just the reverse with me now."
Well, part of the new me insists. Just as I told Anne and Gottlieb
that I wanted some attention to be paid this time. None of this
"what difference does it make, you and I know you're a good
writer, a hundred years from now you'll be Jane Austen." I want
it now. I don't say why, but the blackmail is there—implicit. (Last
sentence is typical. What is the "blackmail" about wanting your
due? What is happening is that I am giving myself permission to
do or expect what I should have been doing or expecting all along.
Question? Is this a result of age and past experience, or the cancer

experience? I suspect the latter. My permission has to come from Mount Sinai at least, right? Enough of this.)

Still in early morning. Depressed from Mrs. Leibman, I go about my day and am dressed, with girdle (new idea on my part), before nine. First time in weeks. By which I see I am better. I decide to sew a rip that has been bugging me for weeks—take out sewing kit, sit down at window, and there ensues the following. The thimble has my grandmother's initials on it. I have a quick dialogue with Jan and Kathy as, moribund, I explain that the thimble is the grandchildren's great-great-grandmother's, i.e., there are ancestors all around us—and then I take them on a quick tour to show what goes back to where, thinking all the while, "Will I have time?" Then, amused (sort of), I look out the window, see the Chrysler Building, my beautiful, art deco, castle-in-the-sky Chrysler Building, and decide I shall do my dying in this room, my eyes on the building. Elapsed time—ten seconds perhaps. Morbid? Me? Not at all. Oh, yes, I also have a little inner monologue with my friend Janet on the subject of the article on stress and its effect on cancer which appeared in *New York* magazine two weeks ago. Then, another cup of coffee, and I sit here. Upright. Normal. Really feeling very upbeat for the first time in a long time—I don't count parties. At parties I have been drinking two fast Scotches at once, and, euphoric at being among people— never mind if they're dull—and in a new setting, and giddy, I have been having an exceedingly good time.

Okay, let's catch up. I have a sheaf of notes, most of them, since they are handwritten, unintelligible. Let me see if I can extract the wisdom—or nonwisdom. In an experiment, the latter is as valid as the former, I suppose. In no order.

Note 1. "I wake up feeling old. My wrists ache—is that going to be the next thing, that I can't type, I won't have it? First time I have felt old. 'Take up your bed and walk.' Never really heard the meaning of that. Jesus cured all right, but the bed came along, didn't it? Live with what you've got?" I am referring to aches and pains here. Not cancer. Cancer during these last weeks has been almost a forgotten entity, except for the times I shivered waiting for test results. That, of course, is the point of my long-winded description of my entry into my day today. That, feeling well for the first time, I am back on the cancer kick. Fleetingly. Milton was wrong. The mind is not only a place in itself, heaven and hell, it is also Woody Allen. It is impossible not to be enchanted.

Note 2 (several weeks old). "Lying in bed—arms ache—lack of circulation? Reading Florida Scott Maxwell (eighty-four-year-old Jungian analyst writing on how it feels to be old—passionate, resentful, aware of the need to juggle sharing the pain and the sorrow with one's loved ones with assurance, usually untrue, that 'everything's fine, today'), I realize I feel old. Never was middle-aged. I lost twenty years these last few weeks. At least that's how I feel now.

"The damp and humidity of these last few weeks doesn't help. When did I ever notice damp before? Never.

"My phone conversations. Never had so many shocking revelations. In part, I guess, because the image on the other end of the telephone wire is of me lying prone and captive—and harmless.

"I feel an overwhelming lassitude. Too much lying around, I guess. Or is everything catching up?"

Present commentary on above. Is it possible that I needed this back business? I sense that I am using it in a way. I bitch, I complain, I take care of myself, I lie down (after surgery, I pushed myself to walk and to get going and really didn't complain—I think—not that there was much to complain of). It's *okay* to do it. It's *normal,* the back, that is. I am sublimating, getting rid of some of the anger I've suppressed. If that is so, the mind/body gain is something. Or is that Mrs. Pollyanna at work again?

Note 3 (also several weeks old). "I am in a constellation of pain. No matter how I turn, or where I put myself, I hurt. I shall give myself a week (turns out to be two or three), and then we'll see." I read a book about a woman of eighty-two who is dying, but who cannot communicate except by eye blinking. She's paralyzed —totally—but the mind is vibrantly alive. "Like me," I think. That Yeats poem—the old man tied to his "raggle taggle," paltry body. Dear me. Dangerous to be able to be an invalid. If I had kids to take care of, a manuscript to finish (strange, I waited until the book was in, if indeed I had anything to do with it), a job to report to—I wouldn't be like this, I know it.

Note 4. "I am practicing pain. So far, I think I'm lousy at it. Jan and Kathy say I have a very high pain threshold and that I really must have a bad back. I don't believe it. I think I'm just giving in to it. Or rather, I can admit it because, again, it's not a cancer pain."

Note 5 (obviously early on). "I'm angry. I have so little time. I shouldn't have to waste it on this. I'm dying."

Present comment. Last sentence shocks me. Do I feel that way now? I don't know. Deep down, I guess so. But over the long haul, not in the present. (Don't kid yourself, friend. I dedicated the book—copyrighted 1976, I note on the copy, so that's when it will come out—to Gottlieb who really begot it with his blank contract and open check. But I put in an acknowledgment the other day—"with love and gratitude to my husband and my daughters and my father"—so that if I am dead when it comes out, they'll see it. I would like to add my friends and Mark too, maybe my brother and sister, and Kim and Polly, but then it would be ridiculous. But I do know what's at the bottom. From infinity and the unknown I want to call out, "I love you all, I loved you all, I would hold you all close," and as I write this, I weep. I know, I know. We're all terminal, only some are a little more terminal than others. 1976. I'd like to see 1984 too. I think. Funny. This is the first time I've had a sense of missing people if. I just want to clutch it all. Hold it close. My books. My grandmother's thimble. My loves. So many of you. (Please note as the pain of the back recedes, etc., etc.)

·   ·

An episode:

I see Jackie Collins and she reports on the Vineyard (they went the weekend we couldn't). Down the line with people. Coming to one friend—"She's a mess." Me—"Why?" To me, this friend is the toughest, most together, self-possessed—I know, I know, I always know better, but . . . Jackie, looking at me surprised—"She lives on Librium." Me—"Why?" Jackie—"How would you like to live with death?" Deathly silence. Does she hear what she said? Seven or eight years since her husband's surgery, I think. Does Vic live on Librium? Need it? Proudly, I think to myself, "Not at all." Anyway with her husband it's different. He's a man—harder not to be functioning totally. And he had a colostomy, I believe. But I think about Vic. Admire him so. He really has struck a perfect balance between caring and solicitude and normalcy. But it surfaces in touching ways. Yesterday Jan reports he called her at the office early in the morning to tell her what a "great time" I had at the Great Neck rained-out barbecue Sunday. Again, fast drinks, people I didn't know who are therefore interesting as all get out, and I ate too much and puffed out and got the hiccups all of which made me look exceedingly bosomy. Which Vic reported with glee to Jan. "Fine thing," she says, "to have your father boasting about your mother's bosom! Especially when you have none yourself!" But then she says what it is. "He was *so* pleased to see you enjoying yourself." I agree. "It must be hard to come home and find your wife stretched out," she goes on to say, and I correct her quickly. "I'm always up when he comes home," and it's true. But she's more accurate than I. In a way I am stretched out, I guess. And so is he—more than I—with his back. Years of it. But it's different, alas, it's different.

And now, for my father. No question my back went out upon his arrival. (In California, Jean, who wanted him to stay all summer, broke out into fever blisters—"first time in years," she reported—the day before he came.) No question, also that I cannot even remember the two weeks he was here, so if a purpose was intended, it served.

But Jean called yesterday, beside herself, because he has gone back to Florida, was met by Zsa Zsa, indicated he would go with her to London. We're worried that he'll get hurt, worried about what kind of woman this is (fifty-nine, glamorous, "in love" with him inside a week?). But I have an added dimension. Anger. Here I'm stopped, and *my father* goes on. I decide not to call him, tell Jan so in the evening and she looks at me in shock. "He's your father," she says, "he's eighty-four, and he's in trouble," and without answering, I walk to the phone. He's not in, but later I get him, and he says nothing about her or going to London, just sounds flat, so we talk nothings, and after I hang up, I realize it's really early for him to be home and maybe he didn't expect my voice, but hers. But I don't feel angry or threatened any more. I just feel like another human being aware that either way, he's in trouble— as well as not in trouble. And it's none of my business.

Connected with chemotherapy, the above? You bet.

July 27. Oliver Wendell Holmes—at ninety: "Death plucks my ears and says, Live, I am coming!"

Back really better. Not even aspirin these last few days. Just a nagging something, like the television commercials.

But the sense of having been lessened still remains, maybe because I have no real work I have to do.

I am becoming a little puzzled about this journal. It started out as a journal of chemotherapy, but, of course, it isn't. It's a journal of how one lives after one is told one has had (get the "ones"! How put-offish can "one" get?) or has cancer. Situation doesn't change much so there isn't very much to say. Only more of the same.

On Thursday the lights went out and I made some notes in the dark. Mostly unintelligible, except phrase "not easy." True. Not easy.

There is a new openness though. I don't know if it is in me, or in other people. My friend Sylvia comes for lunch and as she gets out of the car, dressed in something loose, she says, "Is there anyone here? Or can I leave off my prosthesis?" I am surprised. She looks the same essentially. And it is the first time in fourteen years she has mentioned it. (I remember the date well—a mastectomy the day after New Year's—she was at a party we gave New Year's Eve, knowing, and I was terrified for her then, and remained terrified for months afterwards. But *she* never seemed to mention it.) Now we lunch and I ask if she wants to swim, and tell her how I had planned to tell her to swim suitless while I went off into the woods (I know she hates suits), and wasn't it ridiculous how we had moused around about the subject before. We don't swim—I'm dubious about myself with my back still—but a ghost has been laid. Maybe.

Two days later, two friends come and swim suitless. Vic politely goes off to the house, but neither friend seems particularly anxious to be topped. New style at Fire Island, I have heard—everyone topless. Later Vic comments at how suddenly flat-chested they are, and says wonderingly, "I don't think I could ever relate to a woman without breasts." "That's a terrible thing to say," say I. He showers, and minutes later says, "I didn't make myself clear. I meant she used to look so great." "I know," I say, "it has nothing to do with me." But it has. It latches on to one of my fears. Does he realize it? He may, and he may very well not. But already in my head I have asked to have only a lumpectomy (Ellen's word), and I have freed Vic to have someone else, assuring him I know he loves me and I understand his feelings—"easy"? No. But I might have had the same fantasy reaction under any circumstances. Again, it is good—as with Jackie—that people don't watch their words with me. I guess.

Another vignette. Vic has been in Washington and saw Masters and Johnson on television. Masters stressed the need for communication and offered one method. You say, "I feel," and add just one word, and then talk about that feeling before you both proceed. For instance, says Vic, "I feel—unhappy." My word

—unspoken—is "scared." I point out his words—we are with friends—and mention mine, and before I can pursue his "unhappy," or *he* can, if indeed he wishes to, I am asked, why "scared"? And easily I reel off a list of "scares," including how I felt waiting for bone scan and IVP results. How—is all this out-speaking a sign of health or neurosis? I know, I know. Labeling is wrong. It *feels* healthier to me, but what does it do for other people? It doesn't seem to me to be hurtful or disturbing, but I have to watch. It could also be boring.

Just opened Florida Scott Maxwell—my eighty-four-year-old friend—and she seems contemporary. (That's the major change recently, I think—I no longer feel young. I feel old. Related to people who are more likely to die sooner than later. Temporary, I hope. It doesn't sound like the most optimistic stance in the world.) Anyway the passage begins, "My only fear about death is that it will not come soon enough . . .   please God I die before I lose my independence." But she goes on to say, "If I suffer from my lacks, and I do daily, I also feel elation at what I have become." I understand both feelings. Also now remember another night thought—that the most I can do for those who love me (and whom I love, of course) is not to shut them out. Because the only way you can be free to take up your life after someone close to you dies is if you have no guilt. And the only way you can have no guilt is to feel you have done all, or at least, the best you can.

Christ, how morbid for a sunny day! But how can a journal about cancer be anything but, by definition.

And yet—please believe, gentle reader—the birds are singing, I am now going to hurry down to the pool before anyone comes, and swim like a slightly achy sleek naked seal and love it, and I am going to meet two people Vic doesn't like very much, but has to see, and then we are going out to dinner and the movies, and life is tremendous. Okay?

And tomorrow to chemotherapy (and maybe the neurologist). I really think—or would, if I weren't afraid of old friend evil eye—that *that* I take for granted. No sweat. Grandchildren to come up too. *I am not afraid to be examined tomorrow.* (Only of saying so.)

Series 6

August 5. So far none of the Sissman fear of the needle probing. It really seems to be something I take for granted. As a matter of fact, driving down yesterday from Montefiore, I had a funny thought. What would I have been doing with myself these last eighteen months if I hadn't been so involved with this? It's like being unhappy and going to see a psychiatrist—that hour becomes the thing you "do" for the week. It's a crutch. Some crutch.

Still it raises a question. Would I have written the book if I hadn't somehow been freed? Would I have done it so quickly this spring if I hadn't a sense of time's chariot thundering after me? (L. E. Sissman finally answered my letter, and at length. He had a gall bladder operation in between, hence the delay. A lovely letter, in the course of which he speaks of the "adrenalin" a sense of mortality gives one. I could use some adrenalin at the moment, with perhaps a soupçon less sense of mortality, but then in between books there is always a pit, so maybe the present is no different from the past.)

I can't remember now how I came to bring it up, but I asked Mark about inheritance and cancer, and said I supposed Jan and Kathy might have some fears about it, and how much of a factor was it. This time he brought out a trillion cells being reproduced daily (last time it was billions of blood cells) and pointed out the incredible feat of their being replicated exactly with defective cells usually being rejected, i.e., not fate, but chance, dictating whether you get it or not. (How about breast cancer, I think, but I really don't know about it. Anyway it sounds comforting.) He also got onto a tack I find enchanting—the historical aspects of cancer. The Egyptians had it, the Greeks had a word, etc. Mentally I add it to my list of things I am going to do IF (or WHEN) it becomes more of a factor in my life—study its history, take up TM, go to "death therapy" classes—in other words, try to tame it by going along with what is interesting in it. Seduce the cobra, knowing as soon as your back is turned, it is likely to pounce. Later in the week Kathy comes from Cambridge and I ask her if she ever worries about herself. Never occurred to her, she says, or words to that effect, and I believe her. "What I do feel is that it's in the family, and that surprises me." I don't bring it up with Jan. With Jan sleeping cobras are better left curled. As a matter of fact, I call her at Fire Island some days after they are settled in, and before she will talk to me she says, "Is anything wrong? Do you have anything to tell me?" I say of course not, why does she ask. "I don't know," she says diffidently, "but now I can talk." Alas, my child. That's what comes of not being a Kathy and letting it all out. (I think. How do I know really?)

Also at the first chemotherapy session, I made my first (successful) attempt to influence my care. I tell Mark that I truly do not want to see a neurologist, and he cancels the appointment. But he does point out that he is doing so because he found nothing in my back to indicate that I need one. Still, inside myself, I did take the responsibility.

Another thing we talk about is pain, i.e., my realization of same during the back episode. "But of course you know how to handle it now," I say, and to my surprise, he replies, "No, we don't. Or rather we do, but our hands are tied," and he tells me about the woman at St. Christopher's Hospice in London who gives heroin and cocaine cocktails to terminal patients so that they are both comfortable and alert. But doctors here cannot obtain heroin, even for pilot project purposes. So I decide to write an article about it.

On Thursday, however, I go to the hairdresser and there I

find the current *Good Housekeeping* with a lead article on the very subject written by a Dr. Glick, Stewart Alsop's doctor at NIH. The introduction points out that a similar article was written by Alsop before he died in response to the sufferings of his fellow patients and that it was published last year. Response: apparently nil. Dr. Glick makes the same points as Mark, except that he does not raise the question of why neurosurgeons may do drastic surgery to relieve pain while internists may not even *begin* medication for the same purpose. I decide to start on a letter-writing campaign. First I have to decide whether I shall discuss it with Vic (cause him anxiety?) I do so, and he gives me a couple of names —Dr. Theodore Cooper at HEW, Kennedy because of his health committee (I think myself a mention of his son will be even more useful). I ponder whether to write Betty Ford's doctor. So far I have written the two letters. Hard letters to write because I think they have to be personal to matter. (Funny, I read Carl Rogers's *On Becoming a Person* on Saturday and he makes the same point Erik Erikson made—the more personal the anecdote, the more general the application, and the more meaningful to teller and hearer. That is surely what I believe—else I could not write at all.) What I wonder is, why aren't doctors who have to deal with pain—or turn their heads away from it—screaming for relief? It strikes me as I write that I really don't know anything about it—it may have a placebo effect, for all I know—but still, it seems to me relief of suffering is as important a goal as curing. Not as exciting, or as satisfying, but necessary. (And what am I doing about old people's homes? Nothing. Easier to forget about them now, as, to be truthful, my sister-in-law Mollie, great screamer when Mom was in one, obviously is doing. What happened to her great crusade?)

I smell a faint whiff of crackpot in me. Which I point out in a note I write Sissman in response to his. I wasn't going to reply, but then looking at his letter, he says, "Please do write again," so I do. And tell him of my letter-writing campaign, hoping that he may use his column as a forum. Ah, insidious.

I am also puzzled about the "stylishness" of all of this. Some of it, of course, is that I am noticing the subject and its ramifications, but there is more to it than that. Already in the magazines that piled up in our absence from the apartment for a week, I have taken out and clipped an article on terminal group therapy and another on stress and cancer. *The New Yorker* has an interview with Barbara Bannon of *Publishers Weekly*, and she says the big theme in children's books for the fall is coping with death. What goes on? Is it part of the inward-turning we are all experiencing in reaction to the disillusions of the sixties? Part of the new openness? It can't be that more people are dying. Or maybe it is that the one thing medicine is doing successfully is giving us more notice—we survive our heart attacks to brood about the next, prolong our cancer careers with chemotherapy, surgery, and radiation. Diseases are not so easy to ignore as if we just got sick and died, finis.

Speaking of which—a young woman in the group therapy article says there is a line, and those of us with cancer (still I boggle at that word—who have had, or may have, I must hasten to add, just for my inner record) are on one side, and everyone else is on the other. I did feel set apart. I don't seem to right now. The bad back seemed to mark a dividing line in *that* feeling. But how do other people feel? Anne, my agent, calls to say she has been reading a book—which she is trying to sell—that made her think of me. It is by a forty-two-year-old doctor, "a genius." He is an analyst, a sky diver, a researcher, youngest head of a department of psychiatry in a university ever, etc. He also has had testical cancer and a major heart attack, and the book is about his attempts to come to peace with his mortality. He has left his wife—or rather, forced her to leave him, knowing he has done so in order to hasten what he expects life will accomplish anyway—become, according to his father, a "hippie," and has been writing furiously. He also has three grown sons, so by Mark's genetic clock, he might be assumed to have lived. Anne reads me a dialogue between the doctor and his seventy-nine-year-old healthy lusty father in which the

older man berates him for his current bizarre behavior: "Why?"
he asks. And the son says something to the effect that he had to
die in order to start living again. Anne is impressed. I'm not sure
what it means. It has the sound of Pangloss—everything for the
best—one more way of denying.

Still, it's not the doctor who interests me; it's Anne. She reads
his book, thinks of me. So for her, I am on *that* side of the line.

Vic, I think, does not put me on that side, and, again there
is a delicate balance to be struck with him between sharing and
assault. Example: On Sunday I noticed a black stitch emerging
near my navel. Usually—though a little less lately—I wrap a
towel around my middle when we share a bathroom, clutch my
underwear, something. But I am also getting used to it, and the
scar itself is becoming less blatant. It seems to belong somehow.
It's not offensive, it's in the middle, therefore has symmetry, and
as it fades, it is the color of my nipples, a small aesthetic satisfac-
tion (we adapt to anything, don't we?). So, without prior thought,
I show the stitch to Vic, who withdraws in panic and refuses to
look. He explains it makes him queasy, although he has had no
compunction about scars, hemorrhoids, etc., with me. I have looked
at his massive infected and tubed appendectomy scar for thirty-
seven years. I feel slapped. Ensues a whole inner turmoil. What
will I do if . . . ? I can die, or choose to live, but only if I move
out. Get a divorce. Can I get a divorce on such grounds? I rage.
Naturally we are supposed to go to Helen's for dinner. Why do all
marital quarrels start when you are supposed to go somewhere
among other people? I am silent, murderously so, in the car, and,
finally, Vic puts his hand on mine. "I'm angry," I say, taking my
cue from Masters and Johnson, and seemingly amazed, he asks
why. I tell him, adding, for good measure, his remark about not
relating to women without good breasts. "Oh, balls," he says, "I
didn't mean that. Anyway it has nothing to do with you." I spell
out my angry fantasy. We arrive at Helen's, still talking loudly,
and she says, "Fight on your own time." I get out of the car and
say proudly, "Our first fight in a year and a half," and it probably

is (anyway I never remember). And somehow everything is all right. I don't think I need to get a divorce—if—but I can't show him a black stitch either.

Still, typing it out now, I realize he is probably right. Certainly for him. He wants no reminders of the line between us. He lacks the one quality that is my saving grace—unselective curiosity. I find even cancer fascinating. A black stitch sticking its head out next to my navel is marvelous. How? Why? What does it mean?

A touching letter from my father about a visit to a nursing home—"It is *horrible*," he says. "I hope and I know our children are different, so let's cheer up and forget the whole thing." Zsa Zsa is apparently in Europe; no mention of her since he returned to Florida. "I hope you are all better," he says, "and you look the same and as beautiful as when you called for me at the airport." So that was *his* version, while he was saying, "She's about your age, but she looks a lot younger." Still, how much more open he is, and worried, too, I guess. I sent him a new robe for his birthday yesterday—I figure he can use it, breakfasting alone or not, either way. At the moment I think it would be nice if "not alone." Progress.

For the record—I just remembered that when Mark said he was going on vacation in a few weeks and that my next series will have to be with some other doctor, I felt nothing until I was on the way home. Then ensued a fantasy—the new doctor finds something, they say I need surgery, but how can I have any treatment at all without discussing it first with Mark? I shall wait until he comes back. I don't think even in psychiatric treatment (treatment? I wasn't having treatment—I just talked to Michael every once in a while), I had this dependency. I guess it is truly a matter of life and death here. Wow. Or, oh wow, to be more accurate.

Notes. My Aunt Peggy wore a ring with the motto, "*Noli Timere.*"

In a red notebook I find I have written Sarah Bernhardt's motto: "Even so." Legless, she played *L'Aiglon.* Even so.

I have just read—for the first time—William James's *The Varieties of Religious Experience.* Naïvely, what impresses me most is that it was copyrighted in 1902. You mean, they thought about meditation, life, death, and all those things *then?* Mostly I enjoyed the quotations. A continuance of the Whitman one about his wanting to live with animals, for instance—"They do not lie awake in the dark and weep for their sins." Also, a list of responses to the human condition. Luther, old: "I am utterly weary of life. I pray the Lord will come forthwith and carry me hence." Goethe— 1824: "I will say nothing against the course of my existence. But at bottom it has been nothing but a pain and a burden, and I can affirm that during the whole of my seventy-five years, I have not had four weeks of genuine well-being. It is but the perpetual rolling of a rock that must be raised up again forever." Tolstoy at fifty: "I felt that something had broken within me on which my life had always rested, that I had nothing to hold on to, and that morally my life had stopped."

And so shall I. Cheered.

August 6. The morning news tells of the Hiroshima bomb thirty years ago today, and I get a very wry feeling. I remember the bomb, and I am sure my first feeling was relief that Vic, in the Pacific, would be coming home soon. I was still full of the earlier reports of our discovery of nuclear energy—that a new bright world would dawn—and I was in the country, I think, away from the paper, and so somehow I was spared the earlier reports. It really was not until John Hersey's book that I realized what we had done. And it was a long while after that that I realized that we—I, too—had done, as much as any "good" German. And it was longer yet—Vietnam really—before I realized that we were all indeed "good" Germans, and were as much responsible for Hiroshima as the Germans generally were for Buchenwald. So this morning when I thought of the hundreds of thousands in Hiroshima and Nagasaki who had cancer, developed cancer, lived in fear of cancer, and still live in fear of cancer, for themselves and for their children, I thought that maybe there was a faint, a very faint, hint of justice in my having it. A strange and devastating thought. Not the guilt of doing—after all, I really had no say— but the guilt of judging others who had as much to do with "doing" as I. But then, that presupposes a special Fury watching over me, and then my sin becomes even worse—hubris—and so I have typed that feeling away. The logic of it, that is. There can be no divine doling out of cancer, or any other evil. But the feeling remains, and I wonder. Is it just another version of "what did I do to deserve it?" Another example of free-floating guilt? I don't know. As usual, for the record.

August 10. Two disquieting notes.

On the way to the typewriter, I noticed a wasp on the window. Same wasp I had seen struggling earlier this morning. In the past I would open a window and let caught wasps escape. This time, partly because it is on a nonopening window, but also because of some other inner motivation, I think I shall play kindly god. (Same feeling of power that makes me walk around a group of ants.) And I take the bit of paper I have in my hand and kill it. Quickly.

My friend Jackie has a slipped disc. Or shingles. My first reaction is a wry kind of pleasure. Now she'll know! Horrible. Later, at my party—of which more anon—I make the announcement that she and Bill, orthopedist genius Bill, can't come because. Same hint of smile on most faces. Why? With them I think it's that the shoemaker's family is shoeless. Something like that. But mine is different. I don't like it. But it's a fact. All her trips— Nepal, Africa, Paris, etc.—the one thing I envy.

And a disc—or shingles—is self-limiting. Ellen is disquieting —plumper (cortisone?), verbose (too much codeine)—but that doesn't please me. It scares hell out of me.

Enough.

I must find something to absorb me because without it the inner monologue threatens to take over. Some nights I sleep so fitfully—as though floating on top of sleep—that I can't tell when I'm asleep, and when I'm awake. Either I'm not active enough physically, or I have lost the distinction between daydreaming and night-dreaming. And it's always Topic A. Sometimes I trace my thoughts back. No matter where they begin—G, L, Z—by some convolution, they arrive at A. I don't like that either.

One of the night thoughts has to do with the quality of medical care I have had in my long friends-with-doctors life. Specifically the treatment of my constipation. Occasioned by review of—though not reading of—Dr. Reuben's book on cancer of the colon, among other things, occasioned, he says, by not enough roughage. Cure: bran. Locking the horse for me, I guess. Elsewhere, I had read that one cause of cancer of the colon—they think?—is carcinogenic substances remaining in place too long in one place because of constipation.

I was always constipated. Psychiatric reasons, I decided early on. When I first saw a doctor—a friend, after we were married—he prescribed cathartics. Then I read "Our Common Ailment," a Consumers Union publication, in the forties, and upon advice of the writer, ignored the subject from then on. Until in the sixties I began to have gas pains of such intensity that sometimes they laid me out. Once, more than once, on trips (it was especially difficult on trips—if we were away three weeks, I tended not to evacuate for three weeks, change of water binds me, rather than the reverse), at any rate, a number of times I writhed on the floor all night with pain. Periodically I would be tested for appendicitis. BUT NO ONE DID ANYTHING ABOUT IT. I had a GI series once. Was told I had an extra loop in my bowel where fecal matter collected (this winter, Dr. Ben in nuclear medicine said, "You must have a lot of trouble with gas, you have so much intestine). No one did anything about it, until once, mentioning it to my psychiatrist, he exploded: "For Christ's sake, didn't your doctor ever hear of Colace? Mineral oil?" So I mentioned it to Phil

Erbans, alas, and he did indeed suggest mineral oil. End of problem. Thirty years later. Locking the stable? Question: Why was I
so passive? "Our Common Ailment." Authority, from the Left.
My fault, somehow, for being prone to flatulence.

Does it make me angry? Sure. Is it pertinent? Probably not.
Dr. Reuben's tome may be one more version of "Our Common
Ailment." But still.

Now, the party last night. Secretly celebrating the first anniversary of Vic's successful back surgery and my feeling well
enough to want to have a big party. Old friends, all dressed up,
nice food, bartender to spare Vic the irritation of dispensing liquor
instead of being able to talk. It was a very nice party, and over-all,
I think, there was a sense of it being a kind of victory. And everyone dutifully called this morning to say what a nice party it was.
And last night I slept nearly nine hours—not fitfully.

Tomorrow shot No. 3. End of this series.

And I am nervous about Mark going on vacation. BUT I
WOULDN'T BE NERVOUS IF I WERE THE ONE GOING
AWAY. Figure it out. I can't. Unless it's a reversion to a childhood dream of security—everything, and everyone, stays in place,
no matter where I may go.

This journal is a bit of a snare. It's not only a lightning rod,
it's a detour. It gives my fingers just enough to do so that I don't
face up to writing. Again.

I have to think of a new self to vacation in. A change from
probing into my own psyche. But who shall I be? The only people
I can think of are more miserable than I am. Miserable? How
did that word slip out? I'm not miserable—I'm the way I always
was, only more so, with the other half just as strong.

·   ·

August 14. From Anne Sexton's *The Death Notebooks:*

> Jonah made his living
> inside the belly.
> Mine comes from the exact same place.

> This is my death
> Jonah said out loud,
> and it will profit me to understand it.

I have been depressed on and off for the past weeks. Today I'm not. Why I don't know.

Monday I waited to see Mark, depressed, or rather, flat. (Again it may be the lack of work. It is a strange feeling to wake up with a day stretching ahead of me with nothing, aside from minor chores, that I *have* to do.) I said something about feeling that I'm on a plateau, and apologized, in a sense, for the flatness, lack of eloquence, of these pages. He intimated that that was what it was about. "It's one thing to be told you have cancer, or to start chemotherapy, but it's another to go on . . ." He didn't finish the thought, but I know what he meant, and it changed my mood. Because that *is* the point. Everyone, to some degree or other, can do arias; it's not difficult to rise to an occasion that comes to meet you halfway. But recitative, dailyness, blanks to be filled, there's the rub. (And I never do learn that the cure for the blanks is to get dressed and go out. My spirits never fail to rise when I leave the apartment where I am mulling and just see people. Even in a bus. Or waiting for one—yesterday I saw a poem pasted on the mailbox on Fifty-fifth Street, and its impact was only partly spoiled by the notice on the other side that the poet's address was either a psychiatric hospital, I forget which one, or a North River pier.) And that is what gives it value—its commonplaceness.

It was our last meeting until October. Vacation for him. Maybe even for me. Reading between his lines, I think he is as aware of uncertainties as I am (which is what makes our rapport, I think, in large part). He was talking about chemotherapy and how variable it is (a difference between biology and physics), un-

less one is in a "protocol." "But," he said, "you do try to make it as
regular as possible within limits, so that if you have to turn your
patient over to another doctor . . ." Again, unfinished thought.

He told me about a patient he had seen the day before who
had had heart surgery twice but did not have the breast tumor her
doctor had feared she might have, and how she sat—husband,
silent, behind her—and talked for forty minutes, starting with the
assertion that she lived each day as it came, grateful for it. My
immediate thought was, "Believe it!" And Mark agreed, pointing
out that the more she talked, the more her bitterness at life and
people emerged. It is Mark's theory that people cannot change
themselves very much, that even in crisis (or cancer?) people act
pretty much as they have been conditioned to. I have to believe in
change—or, at least, adaptation. Maybe what I have is an inner
trust in myself (surprise! I didn't know that thought before now)
that I will not so much "behave" as "profit" by trying to "understand." Okay. That's good.

What else? Sharing, I think—the difficulty between knowing
when to be open (a reference to the episode of the black stitch)
and when one is making the other an "emotional garbage pail." I
put it in quotes because I think it was Mrs. Beneker's phrase, not
mine, and that's funny too, because "she" exists in my mind, apart
from me, as do all my ladies who start out being me and then take
off. I don't know the line, any more than I know the answer to
this one—do I metaphorically try to go to Paris for the weekend,
carpe dieming, or live each day as usual? No choice actually—or
at least, a limited one.

This last week or weeks I have been going to Paris a little
more than usual. Nearly forty dollars for a salmon to feed my
company, a decision to fly to Boston to see Kathy for the day instead of driving, which I could well do. Now, why does flying to
Paris express itself in money terms when money is—or should be
—the least? It's the *seeing* Kathy that's important, not how I get
there. But you know, that's not the point. I also did go to see
Kathy before, so maybe the reason there are no great changes is

that my values were always the same, and pretty good. The only difference is that I am a shade (maybe more than a shade) more self-indulgent. (Or sensible?)

Anyway I am trying to plan a trip between chemotherapies in September. And suddenly I wonder about me physically. Not cancer—or even chemotherapy, though maybe I am too offhand about that. (Mark was most interested in Mrs. Ford's statement about her cancer in her television interview. "Did she mention her chemotherapy?" No. "Did she say that's why she was having such careful monitoring?" No, and then I added, "Is that why *I'm* being examined so much? Not for cancer, but for chemotherapy reaction?" "Yes." "After six months, I realize it," I say, and pat his hand. His response—with very little obeisance to the evil eye on my part, I think, in my noting here—was that looking at my huge record, another doctor would have difficulty seeing that I am indeed getting it. I have it a little wrong, but the general idea is that I am tolerating it very well indeed. "Does that mean I will continue to do so?" "Most likely." In this, our life, God wot, there are no certainties, right?) To go back to the trip—Sicily is where I've chosen—suppose I react there? So I do.

More worrisome is my body and its aches and pains. My back hurts slightly now, not enough for aspirin, just enough for me to know it's there. Last night a cramp in my leg woke me. It was gone in a matter of seconds. My wrists ache on and off. I have two feelings about my body, one negative, one positive. The negative —the aches and pains—makes me feel as though I have suddenly and prematurely aged. Now, I am not unique in this. Jackie, younger and laid flat with her disc, is appalled. Everyone seems to have a back or some variant—look at Margit, thirteen years younger. Look at Vic. And so on and so on. But I wonder whether my aches and pains aren't in some way connected. The back certainly came post-surgery. And edema, according to Mark, affects the muscles affecting my wrists. Does edema from chemotherapy pinch the paths of my muscles, and is that what makes me achy?

Will I be able to walk and sightsee and climb as I used to? I can try. I remember all the old ladies on trips; I know now their trouble must have been their aches and pains.

The positive reaction is something else. I keep feeling a little like Darwin's evolutionary hill inside—as though things are going on, a struggle for survival of the fittest, and as though I am winning! Or at least not I, but the independent forces within me. This is not a Pollyanna say-it-so-you-will-believe-it-and-it-will-do-you-good reaction, it is a gut one. I am truly convinced.

What else? The inner monologue? I mentioned it to Ellen, who came over very depressed because she thinks she is getting worse. I said what I truly feel, maybe she is, and maybe she is just on that famous plateau, in part because she is alone so much now and has, like me, only herself to set a framework. And when I mentioned the monologue, she nodded at once in agreement, I didn't even have to spell it out.

Well, middle of the night in the country (for some reason I don't sleep well there, but I do in the city, so, as I thought, it is more a mechanical, outside of myself, thing than a sign of inner turmoil). I thought that if anything happened to Mark, I would transfer to Sloan-Kettering because it would be more convenient for Vic and Jan to visit. From there I got to changing the furniture in the apartment so that I could expire tastefully in the study surrounded by books and gazing out at the lovely Chrysler Building, a completing of the circle from the time I used to watch the towers of New York from my Latin class at Bay Ridge High and think of them as Camelot. In the scene I am both pain-free and palely Victorian, and I even take with equanimity the possibility that Vic can walk easily to see special friends between times spent with me.

I wonder? Do I play these scenes so they *won't* happen?
Maybe.

I also one night woke up angry at my mother. I keep struggling to understand why I felt—feel—no more because of her death. (Writing the last two words gave me a chill. Maybe I don't

acknowledge it—after all, she did live a thousand miles away.)
And something in me—the anger—was saying, "Don't expect me
to feel sorry for you, you had twenty years on me!"

Easy to figure out the connection of what's coming next.
Kathy's memoir on me got sold to *Ms.* incredibly quickly, very
well paid for them—$500. Vic's first reaction was hoots of
laughter (he called me when Lynn called him, unable to get me),
because he knew what my first reaction would be—nose out of
joint. Is there *nothing* she can't do! Was it that, or my unwillingness to be put down as a cancer patient? (How different is it from
the way I've used them? *Very.* Believe me.) Then I became very
pleased, and am increasingly so. I spoke to Kathy and she said
that Lynn said *Ms.* made nothing of the cancer, it was the relationship between mother and daughter and the thoughts on pregnancy
that impressed them. Good. We are all myopic when it comes to
ourselves, I guess.

August 16. Off to Boston. Back, and then to Long Island. In
a way feel as if I'm practicing for a (the?) trip. Not in September,
but maybe in October. For the first time I feel fragile—conscious
of aches and pains—*can* I travel? (The back, not anything else.)

This morning I saw a commentary on Mrs. Ford's famous
interview by Harriet Van Horne and, a psychiatrist, Dr. Erika
Freeman. Van Horne was critical in a snobbish way—she showed
"poor taste," the interviewer asked the questions he did because although she is a dear woman, she is not "very interesting." Freeman
exploding. This woman studied with Martha Graham, she's a
person in her own right, furthermore, I'm tired of the victim being
blamed, the question was rude. Astonishingly Van Horne demurs,
then says, "But we must treat her tenderly, she's been so sick!"

Good Lord! The ultimate snobbery! I react so violently I see
how strongly the line is drawn, and how much I resent it. (Truthfully though I feel it's theoretical with me, internalized anyway,

because I don't *look* or, I think, act it, because, I think, I'm not. End of circle.)

Got Dr. Reuben's book on diet. Decide I will eat bran three times a day. Then realize (a) that I had better ask and (b) that the point of it is to have one's bowels move, and mine do. Mark always inquires about same. Is it because of the Reuben thesis? Since I read the book on Saturday I have had a mild case of the runs. Mind over matter, or a surfeit of tomatoes? Or do I unconsciously—or not so unconsciously—buy wheat and dark breads for myself and actually eat them, I who never used to eat bread or cereals—feed myself differently?

Every morning I wake up with some sentence relating to cancer in my mind. Innocuous mostly, but it makes me wonder about my subconscious. Which is now pressing me to write that I met Bob Bernstein, president of the whole Random House complex, which includes Knopf, Saturday night—first time—my publisher-once-removed—and talked a good deal to him, but never once, so far as I can recall now, thought of myself as having had (or, okay, having) cancer, or being under an obligation somehow to let him know. Don't ask me to explain. Fact.

August 23. Back from Boston, dinner out in New York the next day, traveling to Cutchogue (three hours), Wainscott, Amagansett, Shelter Island, Cutchogue again, swimming, car-riding, sleeping in strange and occasionally uncomfortable beds, sightseeing, long trip back to Mount Kisco, traffic jam Sunday night and a storm, which made the half-hour trip from Larchmont to New York take nearly three in panic, dark, and flood—and I feel better than I have in months and months. No backache, and most of all, no thoughts of cancer, until this morning when I woke up to think that I wasn't waking up with a thought of cancer.

My trip to Paris has been a wild success.

In a real sense it's the first time I've been away since the first surgery—going to Sarasota, after all, was simply going to my own house—and it is astonishing to me how much I needed the change. Not even to be in a hotel, which we weren't—just in another house, in other surroundings. To be among people!

I feel just fine, and a little rueful. Because it suggests that if I were busy all the time I wouldn't have time to brood—if that is what I am doing—but on the other hand, if I were busy all the time (which I can't be), I wouldn't be able to do any work. Assuming that I will be able to get on with it. And, moreover, I would get tired. That I did by Friday afternoon, when we couldn't wait to get back to Cutchogue and peace at Hattie's. BUT that isn't sickness (or knowledge of my friendly local cancer)—Vic was even more tired. And *his* back hurt.

Charles Revson died today. Cancer. And not all his money . . .

I got an answer from the Assistant Secretary of Health and Welfare on my letter about the heroin potion for pain. He thanks me for my "touching and sensitive" note, says he knows nothing about the use of the "anodyne" (lovely word) I mention, but will look into it in the proper places. I hope so.

It strikes me today that what one needs most is trust in oneself. Soma and psyche, both. (I love the "one"; whenever I get Pollyanna philosophical, I lapse into "one.") Hubris, that last statement, I think. What comes to my mind now is a mention Alice Frankel made of a psychiatric patient of hers for whom she had to fill out a German reparations form. She was suffering from a "depression caused by cancer," Alice explained, using the adjective "widespread," or some such, I think in a bit of deference to me. (I keep wondering how "encapsulated" I seem to people. During the Long Island journey I had no sense of encapsulation, or being on another side of the line at all.)

The fact is I feel so normal—not even a back twinge!—that I have to *make* myself write this.

Tomorrow is another day. Alas. I know it. All is flux.

·   ·

August 31. One day before September—and the New Year. Always at this season I feel like a child waiting for school, and a new life, to begin. It is as though the time of waiting is over, and I am going to get to work anew. (I know. I wrote about it once—and better—in *Mrs. Beneker,* but that was about Sumerians and Akkadians. This is about me. Flat. Plain.)

I have been browsing among my bookshelves. Looking for answers or inspirations. Came across the *Science and Health* my sister Jeanie gave me a couple of years ago. I had had a vague idea of reading it through (like Proust, which I *am* going to do) to see whether, indeed, some miracle would occur. (Truth. This is the place for it.) Chapter 1 starts with a quotation on prayer. Jesus on faith moving mountains. It ends with, "Your Father knoweth what things ye have need of, before ye ask Him." Numinous. That was all there was to be said. The rest was commentary, and a mishmash. Some truths, of course. Your arm doesn't move itself; your mind, whatever that is, moves it. Also, a surprising bit about doctors. They should be Christian Scientists, says Mrs. Eddy, because their belief about their patients' conditions influences the patients. No question. Mark conveys to me my health. If he didn't . . .

So much for Christian Science. It's obviously not my thing. But a firm belief that I am well—that I have. Because I have no reason to think otherwise. Not easy to maintain. I have been reading steadily the last weeks since I am not writing, and it seems to me every book I pick up has someone dying of cancer. Even *Point Counterpoint,* which I am now halfway through, is going to have old Bidlake die of stomach cancer; the symptoms have already been laid out. And they all die so horribly! Ugh! And Ellen comes with her symptoms, and Walter Sachs's symptoms—enough. This *is* a journal, not a garbage pail. But I do sometimes have the feeling I am standing on a hilltop, braced against a tree, with a harsh wind doing its best to blow me away from it. (The Tree of Life? I don't know. The image is of me well, but against demons trying to tell me otherwise.)

I had my hair cut off. It is all curls. No upkeep presumably. Vic likes it; everyone at Marian's Friday said at last I had achieved the proper style. I nod and smirk. Two fantasies. One—that I look like Jan at sixteen when she was heavy and curly and had braces on her teeth. I see myself younger, no doubt about it, and half look for braces on my teeth when I look in the mirror. Very positive. But two—if I have to go to the hospital it will be easier to keep my hair in shape. Nuts.

This has been a week of battling the evil eye and, at the moment, it seems to be under control.

First I went to the spa on Fifty-fifth Street to find out if I could swim and pay by the visit. No soap. But I got the price down to about a third if I signed up for the year. Question? Will I use it? Will I have to go to the hospital again? Will I die before the year is up? (What difference if I do? That I never thought of.) But I decided (a) if I am all right, I should be less pudgy (I don't really mind the heaviness so much, it's just that I could be less flabby if I tried), and (b) if I do need surgery I would be in better shape for the exercising. So I wrote out a check and joined. Count one against the evil eye.

Then, at Lynn's, I showed the girls the pictures of Kim and Polly in my talisman locket and the locket broke in two. I DO NOT REGARD IT AS AN OMEN. I shall have it welded together next week. In the eye of cancer, a broken catch is hardly momentous. (Don't ask me why "eye" is always my word. Eye of God? *Sub specie aeternitatis,* if that's what the Latin is? I guess so. What's important and what isn't?)

Most difficult engagement of the week was the visit to social security to see about getting disability. Rationally I think I am entitled. All the arguments—paid in for thirty-eight years, etc.; really couldn't work full-time, etc. But could I, if I had to? I don't know. The back certainly threw me this summer, and I find it hard to get through a complete day without some stop in the afternoon. But if I *had* to? I tell myself it is holier than thou not to apply—I need the money, I would relieve Vic of some burden, it is not up to me to make the decision, etc. But I was uncomfortable. As though I was tempting fate. On the other hand, if you have—had —cancer, and may still have—or again have—cancer, don't you deserve some minor compensations? Still, denial being what it is, I felt I was lying, even when I gave the dates of my surgeries and the fact that I am getting chemotherapy. It was as though saying it made it all real, whereas if it wasn't down—but that's evil eye business, and has nothing to do with my becoming eligible for medicare in two years if I get the disability. (I should live so long! I said it to the woman taking my application, and *that* at least had the ring of truth. It's very possible I won't, and at the same time, I think of myself going on forever, an old lady saying, "Yep, I did indeed have cancer, long, long ago!")

Intimations—from Pamela Hansford Johnson, wife of C. P. Snow, in *Important to Me.*

On having a tumor—found to be benign—removed: "All this brings me, however, to the contemplation of death. Death is a part of life: birth the opening, death the completion. I do not follow Dylan Thomas's rhetoric—'Do not go gentle into that good night' (same feeling I have always had!). My only hope, and I think it is the hope of most people, that I go very gently indeed. But there is always the dread to beset us, of a lingering illness, in great agony."

Contemplating euthanasia: "I think I should have a rather dishonorable hope that he (her doctor) would do so without being asked. Dishonorable, on my part, because I should be laying a dread responsibility on other shoulders. But I doubt if I am capable of the ultimate stoicism."

On mourra seul as Pascal says and which my husband has often quoted.

Not on death—but on Aldous Huxley—"he was my higher education." Mine, too, in a way—with *Point Counterpoint.* Rereading it now, he has a marvelous part about Mozart dying, and his body nourishing lambs and spinach, which in turn go to make other Mozarts. A.H. would turn in his grave at this simplification, but I am not about to look it up. Her Huxley was *Texts and Pretexts,* which she says is unobtainable now. But I have it. Peggy's. One of the books I found in my browsing. Forty-two years old.

"I like the image of a life as a swallow flying in from the darkness into the great hall, and, after its moment of light, out into the darkness again. But if it is to be acceptable to me, the swallow, after the second darkness, must come into the light once more."

(*Timor mortis conturbat me.*)

Few intellectuals have been undisturbed by this. It has a ring to it that is almost a jingle. It could be a song for skipping to:

Eenie, meenie, miney mo,
Timor mortis conturbat me.

I don't know why we all regard death as so peculiarly special. It is the great commonplace. Birth seems much more extraordinary.

My mother—mine, VBW's—left a note in re death saying that no one knows he is being born, or knows where he came from, or worries about it, and isn't the process of dying the same, another birth into where? True—the difference, of course, being that you *know* about death, and presumably don't about birth, and the one is full of pain and indignity, or can be, unless you pop off (in *my* family—mother's that is—they almost did—Grandma, Mother, Ernest, Peggy, even if it was in the hospital, could that be in my genes too? Nope—my genes are on my father's side, I suspect).

At any rate, Johnson ends this bit with: "Meanwhile, it would be as well if I started thinking about writing another novel."

A good place to end this. And to note—elsewhere—about another novel.

Series 7

September 3. Thirty-seventh wedding anniversary. I am a little depressed today, why, I can't tell. Not the anniversary, I think, although all "occasions" have their *tristesse* I have begun to see. A response is expected, and because of the expectation, and the sense of failure to meet that expectation, a kind of resentment ensues. I never was aware of it until I began to understand why Vic resents birthdays and rejects presents and feels uncomfortable with "occasions." He doesn't want to be *made* to feel anything.

But I don't think that's the source of the depression. More not having gotten into any work, I think, so that the days have to be filled impromptu. Nor is the source a realization of another milestone. The electric blanket is that. (And I was happy to buy it yesterday, I realize.) Our blanket went last spring and I forbore buying a new one on sale. Didn't know whether the house—or I —would be around. Well, we both are, not ready to be turned in for new models. Thinking which, this morning I had fantasies of my expiring. Where? In town or in country? Ugh. (I know why. Carryover from—and I even block on her name. The last one I can get—but her first name? My good friend? Alas, the mind! Or is it, how marvelous!)

Vic had a nightmare the other night. I started to put my hand on him and say, "It's all right. I'm here." And then I wondered. Am I the nightmare?

I, too, had a dream. I am in the house of a doctor friend, and he is going into another room to tell his mother-in-law she has cancer. In preparation he is putting on a smile and a pooh-poohing hopeful expression. I stop him. "Is life really worth living?" I ask him. "Can you honestly tell her not to commit suicide?" I get no answer.

What is the foregoing all about?

The absence of my doctor. Dr. Mark Markham. Mark. I am shocked to realize the difference it makes. And my dependency.

I was vaguely uneasy all weekend, as witness the dreams, and fantasies (lots more, all of them on the same subject), and seeing Dr. Bulkin didn't help. Nothing to do with her, I'm sure. Her patients might react the same way if they had to see Mark. At first I was looking forward to having a woman for a doctor. First time. I even made up a little speech I would deliver about it and then of course realized that it was patronizing, and sexist, even to notice the difference. Well, it was different, even in its physical aspects. As it would be if it were a different male doctor, I suppose. But for the first time—well, not the first time, I suppose, it must have been true seeing the other doctors—I felt like a patient. Period. Anonymous. And the chemotherapy seemed more real. (Nagging reminders at the lab in Westchester when the woman taking my blood said my vein was "all scarred" by way of explaining why she hurt; Dr. Bulkin reduced the Alkeran to five tablets because of my platelet count, "perfectly natural, to be expected," she assured me, but still. Reality. With Mark I usually get out feeling somewhat elated; here, I went out into the oncology floor, flat.

I'm not getting it right. I don't know what it is, but it isn't quite what I've been saying. All I know is that Mark's is a hand I hold on to, and when it isn't there, I feel very shaky going over the plank. EVEN THOUGH SHE SAID I WAS DOING VERY WELL AND TO MY REMARK ABOUT WHETHER I DO OR DO NOT HAVE CANCER, SHE SAID, "I GUESS YOU DON'T." Right now, I added to myself.

Do you know what? All this adds up to is how incredibly lucky I am. (Flashback to Kathy saying that, in re my not reacting badly to chemotherapy, and then laughing, "Sure, lucky to have cancer!" But the first is true, too.) How wonderful to have a "meaningful relationship" with my doctor. Trust. And is that what faith-healing is about? Everything ends up in a circle. Zen. There are more things on earth . . . That I believe.

.   .

Freud had twenty-nine operations in sixteen years according to Helene Deutsch, who received a letter from Anna Freud after the twenty-ninth reporting how Freud walked in London and enjoyed the fresh air after the rain. "He accepted his sufferings patiently, and nothing could destroy his capacity to enjoy even the most modest gifts of life."

Not related but:

"All the best human impulses can be traced back to adolescence. I believe these persistent adolescent forces are the best aspect of my old age." Optimism, I think, is one of my adolescent forces, and wonder, and curiosity, all of them *my* best aspect. ("Optimism" is a strange word to use in the face of all my fearful fantasies, but again, I think they are the playing out of the unthinkable in order to be able to cope, not because I think of them as the only reality. As a matter of fact, I am convinced that life always surprises.)

Kathy asked me if I had seen the one great quotation in the Deutsch book and I said I didn't remember it. But I see I wrote it down, to wit: "That person is lonely who has no one for whom he or she is Number One." Amen.

September 9. Funny. Even the journal stands still when Mark is away. Saw Dr. Bulkin yesterday and again it was so different. Hospital hadn't phoned in my blood report, or if it had, no one had it, so we had to wait around while Jane got hold of the lab in Mount Kisco. Dr. Bulkin muttered, "I have to see patients," which, indeed, she did, but it wasn't my fault. I had already been waiting a half hour or so while she went down with another of Dr. Markham's patients to arrange something which later turned out to be a "bone scan," "urgent," "diagnosis breast cancer," all of which I saw on the table in the examining room. Very depressing. It means the nice woman I see occasionally in the office with her husband is having trouble. (On the other hand, I had a bone scan and it was negative, so I shouldn't jump to conclusions. But I should. I know it.) The blood results forthcoming, I got my shots. Period. I don't even think she draws blood, or if she does, she does it remarkably fast. No, she doesn't. There's no red ampule around. Okay. It's not necessary, and we really have nothing to say to her. (Freudian slip—to each other, I meant.)

Still I realize as I leave that I feel somehow diminished. A patient. Needy. Just a holding battle. Destined for that oncology floor. But when I leave Mark's office, I feel good. Expanded. As though we are partners—equals in a sense—in a job that we are doing together, and that we are doing it well. The equality is there along with the paternal, Godlike aspects that are present too, alas. Nothing that Dr. Bulkin does, really. What she says is fine. "You need the medication to keep you well," in response to my asking, woman to woman, what is the best thing to do to keep the hair off my face. I'm not complaining about the medication at all, although that's what she hears. The only time we connect is when I mention swimming and she asks me where I go and tells me she is afraid she will get muscles from the gym she goes to. Much ado. I see that if I saw her often enough—if I were *her* patient—we would have a relationship.

I have gone to the spa twice so far—swam and bicycled, feeling very tired afterward, and muscle-bound. But I sense it's okay. Only instead of getting thinner, I am fatter. Even my winter coat won't button, I discovered. Still I think I shall follow my body's orders and eat—I seem to be nourishing myself like a squirrel piling up nuts against the winter. The only thing I have to guard against is nervous, bored nibbling.

Read a book called *Creative Malady* by Pickering, ordered via the Portchester Library. When it arrived, it turned out to be not quite what I had expected. Fascinating in its insights into Darwin, Nightingale, Eddy, Proust, et al., but Pickering was talking about *psychoneurotic* illness, which is a different horse. Not applicable. Actually I'm in a reverse situation. They felt ill and weren't, and I don't and am. (Maybe.) But at one point he mentions how modern medicine has managed to "cheat death" and for the first time, I got a cold chill. That's what I've done, haven't I? Without the first surgery I probably would be dead now. In another era, I mean. It would have taken over.

Physiological note: I have added bran to my diet and I go to the toilet all day. Probably too much with the Colace.

Am I supposed to have a barium enema this fall? To see Gleidman? I shall wait until Mark comes back to find out. It would be nice not, but . . . maybe the IVP covered the same general territory. My feeling is, don't bother it until it bothers you, but again . . .

Going through old notes, hoping to stir some embers for a novel beginning, I find the following: "Best thing that ever happened to me—Viking's refusal to take the book on old age. (Because I used the material in *Mrs. Beneker*; probably wouldn't even have started on fiction if I had had another adult nonfiction.)" Added comment: "Why *best?* (Why, indeed?) and why, if I think of death, do I only think of an infant book surviving me?"

So I thought of death back in 1969 or 1970!

Saw Jackie last night. Her face terribly distorted still, but it's not Bell's palsy, only a virus which will pass soon. She didn't want to see me, I think, until she found out what it was, because she was embarrassed to be complaining in front of *me* (I think so) and also because we seemed of a pair. Now that the balance is unbalanced again, it's okay—for both of us, actually. I don't think it's paranoia in me, simply realization of a fact. Which is maybe why I spoke of going up to Montefiore and chemotherapy and the difference in doctors in a very flat, matter of fact, factual tone. I don't usually, but I had a desire to set the record straight. I'm not really different. The situation is quite ordinary.

The day's dilemma—I need a winter coat. Shall I get a halfway decent one, or simply one that will cover me for a few months? Hattie answers the unspoken question when I mention going to look for one with her own version of the right answer: "You should go to Sicily and you should come with me to Sam Wernicke (her 'little wholesale' man). You ought to have what you want." Because my days are numbered? But you can argue the reverse because they are, or even more, because they aren't—why be greedy? I think I'll go to Sam. Cut-rate, but better. Best of all possible worlds.

Thus does philosophy get reduced to another hunk of cheese and a better grade of mohair.

(Footnote: I settled the winter coat dilemma by going to Abels in Mount Kisco and getting an inexpensive one. The reason, though, was positive. I realized I was trying to get a coat for all seasons. What I need is two—a something to keep the chill out while marketing and such, and a good-looking spring one. Come spring, I shall get the spring one. I can wait.)

September 14. More swimming and riding the bike—up to one mile (like draining the ocean by the teaspoon)—and it seems to me I'm appreciably stronger. Cooked and did errands all day Friday, cooked yesterday, worked this morning, no resting, fine. Hm.

On miracles:

I read about Mother Seton and her miracles the other day and thought, well, why not? How about it, Mother Seton? I asked. No answer.

But just now I read in the *Times* magazine about her canonization, looked at the clock and saw it had just begun. So I ran to the TV, turned it on, and found that only Channel 4 would not work. I ran upstairs, looked at Margit's for a while, came down, turned ours on again. No soap. I just went up, then down, and without looking (but thinking, okay, Mother Seton, do it) turned it on. Glorious living color from Rome. I choked up. Commercial-

ism, Papal politics, long-winded old man dissertation, the Pope being a cannibal eating the communion wafer and wine—all the
same, I wept. My tears are very rare; these just came. Let me not
die of cancer, Mother Seton, I thought (you don't have to say it,
remember, your Father knows!), or, at least, not now. Ten years,
give me. Let me be an old lady. Let Vic be old. Or not have to see
it. I cry some more. All over the world, people are watching; all
over the world, despite themselves, some people are asking for
miracles. "A woman born to love," the article says of Mother
Seton, an imperfect lady ("Most of us treat our defects as guests
at our dinner table. The saints try to put them out"), but full of
guts. "I see Death grinning in the pot every morning . . . and I
grin back." "It seems to me," says the *Times* writer, a woman and
a Catholic, "the search for a saint is nothing more (or less) than
the search for God." What is the search for a miracle? A search
for something that makes sense—value—out of it all. A search
for strength to climb the mountain.

I run around the driveway five or six times until I get too
breathless. I swim. I ride the nailed-down bike. A search for
strength. Amen.

September 16. Said farewell to Dr. Bulkin on Monday.
Awoke fitfully Sunday night, realized it was a shade of anxiety
over seeing her. But there was a very casual examination ("I'm
not going to do a pelvic," she said, "I'm satisfied with what I found
last time"), and she was very amiable. "Keep well," she said when
I left, and that's about it. We're in a holding pattern. The only
uncertainty is how long. Which, of course, is true for everyone.
What else is new?

(Spent last night—Yom Kippur night—with Abe and
Frances. Strange in a way, because they are so anti-Israel and pro-
Arab. We talked about it, managed to keep above anger or hurt.
In a paradigm of the Jew-Arab relationship, something had come
up before about planning. What? Oh, yes. About teaching. I said,

as always, that I would like to but I didn't want to take on any responsibility. That's true. The thought of committing myself a year ahead is appalling. Was it when I wasn't—say, uncertain? Yes. I didn't do it before either. But I had an external reason then too. Or do I look for them? I could just as well have committed "because," as the reverse. Anyway both of them looked at me and asked, "Why not?" knowing full well the answer. "Well," I said, "knowing that Frances was there before, if she isn't now, and I guess she isn't, fourteen or fifteen years of grace is a rather convincing time. There's this long corridor, you see. With a door at the end. Everyone sees it, but for me the door looks much closer suddenly." "But that's true of everyone," said Abe, and I said, "Yes, but for me it's more so." With no heat or emotion. Fact. But I wonder now how much I ascribe to the cancer, and how much is age. I never think of age as a factor. Never did. Never think of myself as anything but middle-aged, if that. I sit on myself to keep from getting up and offering my seat in the bus to gray-haired ladies, forgetting that there but for the grace of L'Oréal . . . Jane was saying how tired she gets, and how serene she is in some ways too. "Getting older," she explained. Hattie complains of fatigue. "I just can't do what I used to." If I get tired, I assume it's postsurgical.)

We went to Nantucket. Going away, as usual, was a release and, as usual, even when the plane was coming in after a stormy flight, I was sorry for it to land. When we're away, it's as though we were in a cocoon, safe. Or is it that I'm not writing, and when I'm away I don't have to feel guilty about it? And that Vic is around? This time the pang didn't last very long, though. It was nice to get back to the nice dry serene apartment after the beginning-to-be-soggy cramped guest house room.

Several things about Nantucket. First, the pattern was startling, or would have been, except that I have come to take patterns for granted. Last time, I was there with the Bernsteins. Alone. Where Vic was I didn't know. She was recovering from her cancer surgery. And I said—I don't remember it, but Frances has, and mentioned it several times, the last time only a month or so ago, when she said, "Do you still feel that way?" and when I said, "Yes," she said, "Good for you!"—anyway, what I said, and surely felt, was that I envied her, loved, caring, and cared for and would have gladly swapped. So there I was—the swap, in a sense accomplished, and doubly cared for, because Jan and Lester were along too. Caring and cared for, and together. And Vic, who I never would have thought would enjoy the history and the quaintness of the place reacting just as I had. It was a different place for me this time, of course. The novel began there, and I checked what I had written against the fact of the locale. Accurate enough, but I never would be able to write it now. Ancient history. Someone else. Different island.

Add to patterns—the first evening the chimes in the Congregational church led off with the hymn, a Christian Science hymn, sung to me every night of my childhood by my mother when she got me to bed.

And the plane, befogged at leaving, took off when the skies cleared suddenly, ran into a storm at New Bedford, landed and took off again with not one, but two, rainbows in the sky. Rainbows I always take as a personal message. I hunt them down as soon as I glimpse a juxtaposition of sun and cloud. I think I bagged one a couple of months ago over the Pepsi-Cola sign looking out of the living room window.

Off pattern—and perhaps more significant—is that this is the first time since the first surgery (that phrase is almost Victorian in its evasiveness, isn't it?) that I haven't come back with a sheaf of notes attesting to a preoccupation with noting what I was thinking. That's silly. What I mean is, usually I take notes that have something to do with me and cancer. But this time I didn't think of it except in the two late afternoons when everyone was exhausted from too much walking, and Jan said "I don't know how you stand it, I'm so tired I can't make it," and Vic said I had to rest. And I did, for a couple of hours each time. (As I would have had to anyway probably. As did Vic.) What I thought of again was Louise Doonieff's poignant remark—"You'll find that one of the pluses is how wonderful it feels to rest."

BUT THAT WAS ALL. I felt very strong, stronger, I should say, probably from the exercise I've been doing. I'm flatter too. Just as heavy, but my pants close.

I also realized that since I started thinking about a book— maybe that's why—I don't think about cancer so much. I also have not been waking up with it as my first thought. Now, like the character told not to put beans up his nose, I sometimes think, "Look, Ma, I'm not thinking about cancer!" But it's true. The passage of time? Getting used to it? Having to push to feel it because I really don't feel any different? I don't know. It doesn't seem so much of an *idée fixe*. Or maybe it's one that's so established I don't bump into it all the time. Surely when Jan and Les talked about when they would be going back, or rather going back to Nantucket, I could see the door at the end of the corridor. And when Jan said Kathy and her husband Hilary hope some day to get a house there, I thought to myself that it was too bad I wouldn't be around to see it.

A casual thought, though. No emotion to it. That's how it is. (But I'm going to fool Fate, am I not?)

Last night in bed I thought about what I ought to write. First about Louise Doonieff. Don't combine the two books, Louise and Peggy. I always do that. Like this last one. I had to get my father and grandmother in because I didn't think I would have the chance to do them later. Failure of nerve. Louise gives me a chance for anger, and for sickness. The next one should be Peggy—all passion spent, how to live with it gallantly, a dying book. (Maybe I won't be ready for it then, either.) The last one should be this. So then I thought of how it should begin—the anecdote about my grandmother and how she was afraid of dying and how I lectured her (at twenty) and read her Cicero's *De Senectute* to induce stoicism, and how she listened unconvinced, and then I got a mild case of sunstroke, and called her in the middle of the night, and said, "Grandma, I'm dying," and she asked quietly, "How do you like it?" I didn't like it then, and I don't now, is what I will write. A good beginning. Then I thought of Keats and the line, "Now more than ever seems it rich to die,/To cease upon the midnight with no pain." Wasted on fifteen-year-olds. I didn't understand it until this minute. To have tuberculosis, and know you will die, and to have the wish to "cease" with "*no pain!*" Of course.

Enough of this, and my excuse to avoid beginning.

My Father's Flu

September 26. Very disturbed. The afternoon I wrote about our return from Nantucket—everything calm and under control —I got a call from a woman saying my father was very sick, a virus, with high fever; that she had been caring for him for days (who was she? where did he meet her? No idea. I thought she said her name was "Kelly" something, but it turned out later, speaking to Jean, that it's "Tilly," and that she is a friend of Aunt Ethel's. Jewish, in other words, not the red-headed Irish lady I quickly made up in my mind), and that she was "very tired." Implication—I should come down. Yes, he had seen the doctor, he was on antibiotics, the doctor had suggested he go to the hospital if there was no one to care for him, but didn't feel it was necessary otherwise.

My back against the wall. (As it is now, when it's out of my responsibility.) As far as I could tell, it was a simple virus—the doctor had said he didn't think the antibiotics would do much— and my father sounded fair, if upset, when Tilly put him on the phone. The main thing was that I had not yet called him—I had told him I wouldn't call on Sunday because I would be away, but he forgot—and my sister Jean hadn't called him (turned out she had overslept and had a class Monday morning), and he felt deserted. Taking a deep breath, I explained to Tilly why I couldn't come down unless it was an absolute crisis—which she agreed it wasn't. "Oh, I didn't know," she said, "does your father?" I said he did, but he wouldn't let it register.

I called at night, he sounded better, Tilly said she would go home. Next morning she was still there, but he now had no fever. It seemed to me what he needed was a visiting nurse or companion, and I got hold of the Hollywood, Florida, yellow pages. Sure enough there was a whole page of bonded, by the day or night aides and nurses who would be available so I called back, gave Tilly the numbers, told Dad he ought to have someone stay the night, he said weakly, "Whatever you say," and I thought that was that.

Then I talked to Jean. Yes, she had ("with my fingers crossed") volunteered to go to Florida, but "Dad said no." Also, she would be glad still to have him come live near her in California. She thought it would work out fine.

My reaction? As usual, I am consumed with guilt. I think I am *using* the cancer in a despicable way. Because the fact is that this week I can go down—I'm not having shots. (Jean kept saying she wished I weren't having them, "ask them to stop," she said. Christian Science.) BUT I DON'T WANT TO, AND I WOULDN'T EVEN IF I DIDN'T HAVE—WHAT? THE EXCUSE? I mutter about my white count, and that I shouldn't be near contagion (true? who knows? no one said anything about it, it's just bits I've read which probably don't apply, because my white count is okay obviously). I also wonder whether I am physically up to it. I *do* lead a very careful life. If I walk around too much, or do too much (what is too much?), my back and leg hurt and I feel tired. (It's the back really that pops up to bother me, nothing else.) I generally lie down when I come in from marketing and carrying big shopping bags, etc. Not for long, but generally in between activity. After swimming, for instance, I have to rest. So maybe it *would* be too much physically. I just don't

know. If I really *wanted* to . . . if it were Vic . . . when it was
Vic (but then I had Margit, didn't I?).

What the block is though—and I know it—is psychological.
As is Dad's need. He said it isn't a physical crisis (as it turned out
he wouldn't have a nurse or an aide or a companion, he didn't
want "a stranger"), but a psychological one. Well, he's eighty-
four. He's entitled. On the other hand, he is a stubborn, difficult
man. He wants to be independent, he knows he's better off where
he is, and that's where he wants to be, but he won't spend the
money to be taken care of. He wants it both ways. Well, he's an
old man, and as with my mother, belatedly I react to his grasping.
(Are you grasping when you have a fever? Maybe. Lots of people
must be alone when they're sick. Without a Tilly to move in and
take over.)

But the fact is that his apartment is a terror for me. I spent
too many anguished, terrified nights on that couch, afraid to be
trapped there, wondering what would happen to Mother during
the night, wondering where Vic was (or wasn't, as it turned out).
I know. I ran down there each time I got a call for my own needs
as well as theirs. More probably. It felt good to be noble, to be
needed, to be the "good daughter." And I needed a place to *go*
where I was needed, and wanted, during those few years, even
though I didn't realize it. But as soon as I realized what was *really*
going on—in my life more than in theirs—I was repelled and
horrified. I DIDN'T WANT TO BE THERE. EVER.

So here I am. Angry. Shaking. Why? Since I haven't had to
go, why don't I just feel grateful, not guilty?

I feel the way I did when I applied for disability. As if I am
using it—cheating—AND I AM GOING TO BE PUNISHED.

I am, please understand, writing this to find out. I don't
know what is coming out as I type. The last is new. I AM GOING
TO BE PUNISHED. Maybe that is the reason for the panic. It's not
really concern for Dad. I assume he's really okay. He has a touch
of flu, the fever is down, he'll be weak, he'll be okay. It would be

nice for his ego if we all ran down . . . okay, okay. Let me reverse it. He calls, I react, I go to Florida. Then what? I can't
picture it because my desire not to go is like a huge stone pulling
me under. The metaphor—drawn from Virginia Woolf filling
her pockets with stones before she walked into the river to drown
herself. I really am angry at myself. Am *I* punishing myself?

I suddenly feel tearful. I say to myself, "Forgive yourself."

Well, all right. No self-pity, but it hasn't been the *very* best
of all possible worlds, has it, kid? So—if without hurting anyone I
use it to protect myself (or to go back to disability—to collect two
years earlier—when I may never live to collect beyond that very
much, after paying in for forty years—anyway, I'm not deciding,
they are—Ellen has no qualms, and she's still on salary, and getting insurance payments, and doesn't have to pay medical bills—
and Vic needs it. I would be stuffy not to try)—oh, nuts, what
would it be like if I didn't have the cancer excuse?

Same anger and terror, and there would be nothing I could
do about it. As a matter of fact, there was a kind of relief when I
heard the diagnosis (I'm kind of making this up, I don't remember
that, but the feeling has been persistent)—I don't have to be
responsible any more.

I think they blame (Freudian slip—I mean I think *I* blame
—and I use "they" as if Mother were still alive!), I think I blame
them for coming between Vic and me, making me put them ahead
of him in terms of presence . . . and that's projection, I know. I
did what I wanted to do. I didn't do all that much. Sometimes,
alas, he encouraged me to go. And now I've written myself into a
stew again.

I have to think about one thing.

IS ALL THIS SELF-PUNISHMENT? And do I deserve it?

If I remove myself—look at me as if I'm someone else—I
would have to say my attitude is the only sensible one. As long as
you can get away with it, do. Why not? . . . I know. "*Get away
with it.*"

The fact is I don't feel I have cancer. (I don't.) So if I use it,

I am faking. And what happens to fakers? They get punished.

I box myself in, don't I?

My stitches suddenly ache.

I shall go and call and see how he survived the night.

He did have a practical nurse. His fever is down to 99. He is going to the hospital. He is so upset he can't talk. Tilly is back. Alas. Alas. He said, "I put up such a fight, and now . . ." He sounds the way Mother used to. She would fight to stay out of the hospital and destroy herself in the process. That's what he's been doing. If he had gone in in the first place . . . it's something we're going to have to work out. (I have a feeling I am going to have to go down there anyway. I don't know. Maybe it isn't as simple as I'm trying to make it. And next week is Jean's one vacation so she can't do it.)

What is terrifying in all the above, I see, is that I have no compassion. I'm not thinking of him, alone, frightened, a bad patient, as always, crumpling into childhood. I'm thinking of me. It's an affront to me. To be bothered. To be upset out of the calm pattern of my days. *I cannot feel sorry for someone who has lived to be eighty-four with no pain, as he himself said, until last year when Mother died.* I cannot feel sorry for a man who is in good health at eighty-four and who always managed to have someone around to pick up the pieces for him.

Something has happened to me in these last years. (I think it was before the surgery, but I'm not sure.) My circle has become very small. I guard myself. (It comes out more so in these pages, of course, because it is a journal of *me*, but even so . . .) There is nothing I wouldn't do for Vic and the children and the grand-children and a few others, but . . . And I am hard. That's the way things are. Tough. If you get old, you will be sick sometimes. That's the way it is. I do not eat my heart out about it. I just don't want to be bothered unless it's necessary—and my definition of necessary is very cold indeed.

I have gone back to my childhood when my love for him was mixed with fear and anger.

On the other hand, Bill Collins loved his father with an uncomplicated, even affection—and he, too, was calm. But caring. I'm not. Is it a displacement of my anger at being more likely to die than he is, younger though I am? Possible. (I don't like these pages, but they're part of the bargain. Truth. Do I need psychiatry? I don't think so. That's how it is. Fact. Would I have wept for Mother if I had not had a cancer operation three months before? I hope so. I weep a little now. But I'll never know. Or is it that even now, dead, she is in many ways more alive for me than he is? A presence. Mother. Please help me!) . . . Help me how? To be more loving. More outward. I don't like this hard ego in the room with me. It's a companion I'm uncomfortable with. Go. Shoo!

Talked to Hattie, so like me that now, in bed with flu, she says, "The only good thing is Joey is in Dallas, so I don't have to feel bad about bothering him." Her mother, in bed with her stroke upstairs. "Do you ever feel resentful?" I ask, knowing the answer. But she goes on to point out some differences. She's the only child. Her mother served her all her life, and helped her through the impossible. But my parents had each other. It is time I faced that the demands were excessive. I make my speech about it being hard to feel sorry for an eighty-four-year-old, etc., and she says, "That's a watershed. For you to be able to say that alone is worth a dozen years of psychiatry." Is it? We talk some more, and somehow putting words into the air to someone is more meaningful than putting them down here, helpful though you are, my beloved Royal friend. I tell her the one great anger I have for the past. She acknowledges it, accepts it, hears it as completely reasonable. Then she points out I am postulating a "deathbed scene," i.e., greater need, when I will be there. "But it's not necessary for you to be there. Ever. You've been there. Many times." Not wholly true, but I see how she has perceived it all these years.

Anyway I feel better. (I! Not my father who is enroute to

the hospital. Still I. Please note.) As though I have learned some-thing, although what it is I am not yet quite sure.

(Footnote: I think his bad patient-ness—and he is, that he is, I'm sure—scares me too. I am judgmental and then think, but how will I be? Will my judgment come to haunt me? Oh, dear, the webs we weave. What I want to be is a joy to everyone, an uplift for the nurses, a miracle to the doctors, a source of abiding love and enduring philosophy for family and friends, my halo a source of warmth and gratification to the entire world (and me, feeling no pain, just a faint Victorian pallor). A gentlewoman's guide to expiration. Ha!

Night. Vic called before going to his meeting to say that if I wanted to go down, he would go with me.

I said no. Located Dad in the hospital. He sounds as beaming as a man can be with a virus. Tilly still there. "Nurses love him," private room, lots of attention. "Relax," says she.

I relax. Find myself thinking it would be nice to be taking care of him, making him feel well, and I laugh. The snake curls back on itself.

No wonder Oedipus tore out his eyes.

September 28. Sunday. Sun shining after the flood and the calm after the storm should be reassuring. But it isn't. I'm un-easy, jumpy, depressed, hoarse. I've been getting hoarser all week. At first I thought it was all the rain, but I'm just as hoarse now. Nerves apparently.

I'm going down to Florida tomorrow. Back Thursday, I hope. I say, I hope, to be on the safe side but actually I know it's some-thing I'm going to have to do. Thank God I have the lab. (Thank God for a little cancer, right?)

In the first place, all the telephoning and talking and agoniz-ing seem to be just as disconcerting as going down there would have been. At least so I think. I may be wrong. Then I know I can do it. It just feels too fake to me to hide behind "my condition," so I won't, even though Bill Collins, who has done his share of running to Florida, says I'll feel like a limp rag and I won't be able to do any good, and if he were my doctor, he'd forbid it. Well, maybe Mark will forbid me to do it in the future. But right now, with only me to judge, I feel as if I have to go. This one time. To try to set things up so I don't have to go again. Easier if he's in the hospital, I think. Anyway I shall see. When Mother was sick, I really didn't feel as if I could cope; now I do, and I'd have little self-respect if I didn't go—what? Big deal. Going in a plane, going to the hospital . . . The problem is taking over, arguing, making him see he has to have help, but on that I feel ruthless. How I'll be in actuality I don't know. He's supposed to be better; that should make it easier.

Yesterday when I decided I would go (leaving Vic doesn't seem to be a factor, maybe that ghost has been laid), I did feel better. Or was it that the Collinses came to dinner to take my mind off it? I don't know.

Kath is depressing too. Feverish, with flu, vaginal infections, Hilary's blood showing her six-month low-cholesterol diet has left her badly anemic—and only yesterday Hilary was telling me how joyous Kathy is in all the work she is doing, fabulously liked as a teacher, better with her patients, etc. Overnight, phft! And she thinks she might be pregnant, so the antibiotics—for strep throat —and the Tylenol for fever may be harmful . . . "intermittent use of aspirin can lead to stillbirth," says she; "whether to have strep or antibiotics is fifty-fifty bad for a fetus" . . . she may not be pregnant at all. She says, "I know I take everything the hard way, make difficult what should be joyous." But the fact is everyone worries one way or another about pregnancy—if you don't want to be, that you are (or so it used to be), and if you want to be, that you're not, and if you want to be, and are, that it's not going to be perfect. Nothing new. I can't tell her not to worry, only that it was always so, and that statistically, most babies are fine. But it makes me sad.

She also says what Vic says—Dad has to make up his mind. If he wants family when he's sick, he has to live with Jean, or near her; if not, he has to be willing to hire strangers. Easy to say, for me too. But his whole way of life is so different. I will have to use blackmail—blackmail when I don't go, blackmail when I do. (I'm being too hard on myself, I think.)

In short, what bothers me is that I want life to be serene. This was to be a good week—another trip to Paris—two theaters, dinner out, overnight at Rhinebeck, a visit with the Fabers. I'll make some of it (I hope . . . I must). But you can't plan. (I started to write, too.) That's how it is. Life intrudes.

Have to write a condolence note to Charles Moos about Vera, dead in an instant of a massive stroke in Nice, returning from "the best vacation ever" in Greece. Bad for him; good for her. Fatuous to tell him so, but seems to me one of life's blessings. Promise me death in minutes after a trip to Delphi, and I'll buy it immediately. Sometimes I think this waiting for the shoe to fall (mental image—large bronzed shoe hanging in the heavens like a star, decade after decade after decade) is the biggest strain of all. Maybe it comes as a relief when it finally bangs down—or maybe that's what giving up consists of, maybe that's when it returns, when your arm gets tired of holding the shoe up there (that's the other image—you have to help the shoe stay in place—the other side of having to be in control, the conviction that you have a say in the matter, that what you do, and feel, counts. But it does, and that's why I resent being impinged upon by Dad's illness, and must acknowledge—for my own self-respect—that it really *isn't* more than I can take. Hubris, hubris, my girl, what an Ego we have there. Good. I respect that).

Talk with Helen about my new cold-heartedness. She nods. Me too, she says. "I have less patience with people," she says, echoing Mark months ago. I spell out why. She nods again. "Does it bother you to have me talk frankly?" "It would bother me if you didn't," she says, and it would. Again, Mark's definition of love. Daring to say, "This is what I am like," knowing it will be heard, and accepted. But then—only partly playing to the gallery and saying what is self-serving—I point out the pluses. "Everything is heightened in way," I say, and I tell her Sissman's remark about the "adrenalin" illness gives you (I fudge, the word wasn't illness, but it wasn't cancer either). "I'll bet you see things differently," she says, and then surprisingly she remarks, "The way you were with menopause," and I am moved. Because she does remember right. It *was* an adventure, super-adolescence, with a little of the wonder of that first-feathered-bird-in-the-hand feeling that the books say you have with the first moving of the unborn child in your womb. A surprisingly accurate poetic description.

Is there a poetry in cancer? Hard to see. I remember suddenly interviewing the Montefiore surgery chief (always block out his name) before Gleidman, and how he said he would take cancer before heart disease any day—"can do more about it." But how did he die? Instantly. Moral? None.

(Night vignette—in the interest of skeletal truth. Replaying surgery and tests, ending with new surgery—mastectomy, colostomy, something unpleasant. Thinking how unattractive I will be, shuddering, turning, and touching a shoulder—carpe diem, I think, while I'm still able to, before I'm repulsive. There are many preludes to love-making, even bitter ones—well, better than anger, or boredom—and what a creature is man, at that, how fast the libido takes over, and banishes the demons—for a while. . . .)

From a Sunday *Times* review of a 400-page personal history and investigative report of breast cancer by Rose Kushner (on the second page, amazingly, a page long)—victim and researcher— "she has tirelessly traveled the globe to bag leading cancer specialists in their lairs." Reviewer very admiring of her to have produced this book—"with scarcely a moment's pause for pain or resignation"—a year after her surgery. Well, yes. And Bickel finished his book a week before he died of cancer. And Ulysses Grant a day before, if I remember. Lucky to be able to do it. Not gallantry. Survival. But what strikes me most is the statistics. *Only* 62 percent survive the first five years, says the reviewer and Kushner; only 50 percent, ten. Implication—failure. But the odds seem awfully good to me. Five years! Fifty-fifty, ten! I realize I think of the odds as 100 percent deep down, while, at the same time, I assume that if there is any deviation, I'll be on the winning side. I just want more time—*off* the cross, whole. Living to be a terror to my aging children isn't a consummation wildly to be desired either.

Just realize I've blocked out the most significant quotation in the review: "Television talk shows and the worry about being appealing not withstanding, the single biggest psychological adjustment a woman must make is to the sudden knowledge that she has a chronic, potentially fatal disease and that removing the breast is only the first step in trying to stop the malignant spread."

Well, yes.

Gleidman said the same thing—"a chronic disease, like emphysema." In the head, that is, for me anyway, nowhere else. Ellen says she'd rather have cancer than be fat. I ask her how fat she is. One hundred thirty pounds. Same as me. I'd take being fatter. Much fatter.

A stitch hurts. Has all week.

Lord make me merry and loving. Forget everything else. Just make me appreciate each day as it comes. And envy my good luck, as that fortune cookie said.

I forgot about Jeanie. We talked about our guilts yesterday —me, for my resentment; she, because Christian Science isn't helping her, or rather, she isn't being a good Christian Scientist and "coping with my first biggie." She's afraid to fly to Florida, afraid to be alone in the apartment, afraid to drive to the hospital. Not to take care of him, if he can be brought close to her home, but he can't. We both feel better. I think. For a while.

. .

October 5. Morning started out like Bad Day at Black Rock —hair on my face (though I removed it Wednesday), an unimportant little fox that nevertheless nips; anger at my father for overturning all my best-laid plans; a list of calls to be made, etc., etc. Now—noon—all is calm again. I spoke to my father, he sounds okay, he will get to California by arrangements made perfectly easily (without me? impossible?), and I realize anew that somewhere I am projecting something onto him, and that even though I say I don't want to be responsible, taking a back seat unnerves me. Of which more later.

The important matter now is that Kathy *is* pregnant. She announced it Friday with awe and joy, and my first reaction was a kind of superstitious gasp that it is working exactly as she had planned (plans again), i.e., she got pregnant right off the bat, just as she wanted, so she can finish her year of teaching and Hilary can take off his third year of residency to concentrate on the baby. My second was, tuned into her, "I'm going to make it." Baby is due in May. No matter what, I should be around then. But to make it until the baby is twenty, grown? Never. On the other hand, Kim is ten, so there's a chance of being around for an adolescent grandchild (tuned into my parents who had such joy of their grown-up grandchildren). All in all, a very flat reaction because the event underlines my limits.

Hours later, I do a double-take. I suddenly think, "I'm a grandmother." And I am very happy. I never felt very grandmotherly about Kim and Polly somehow. They're *sui generis*—Kim and Polly. Maybe you learn to be a grandparent, as you learn to be a parent. By doing. Anyway I feel very ancestorish—and also very motherish about Kathy. Her driving to Wellesley in the snow, her resting (she is anemic, flu-ish, tired), etc. I don't remember feeling that way about Jan, and then it all comes back. Again I've suppressed. Those two pregnancies! The anxiety about her having been X-rayed before she knew she was pregnant; her exposure to Kathy's strange disease, etc., etc. A baby. To be able to hold another one!

I held off until this morning and then called with all my motherish advice, and Kathy loved it. This is my chicken-soup child. She laps it all up.

Back to my father. Yang and Yin. Until he overturned all my goddamned precious brilliant arrangements, it worked out just fine. I got there; found, as I should have known, that he had everything under control. We really communicated very little, mostly because I had to wear the plastic mask, and also because if I got at all serious, he got weepy. I did get him to agree that I could make any arrangements that seemed right to me. His doctor said he was doing well, that he didn't need anyone to stay with him, that he would arrange for a visiting nurse, that all he needed was someone to fix his meals. The nurses, however, agreed he needed someone at night because "the doctor doesn't see him when he falls apart." "Okay," said the doctor, "get him a baby-sitter. Try the boys from the Bible College." I became very angry yesterday when I found that the doctor reportedly now said that he needed full-time care, that it was important he be with family because "they owed it to him," and that he could fly to California on Tuesday if that's what he wanted to do. (Dad earlier had said he didn't want to do that, and the doctor had said he couldn't travel. Who knows?) After my first anger, I realized it was probably Dad putting into the doctor's mouth what *he* had decided, just as earlier he told me the doctor had walked in and said, "All right, you'll live," which the nurses said just wasn't so. In other words, he does what he wants to do, and takes good care of himself. I was also troubled because of Jean, but it turns out everything is arranged. Mark, my nephew, flew down, will stay till Tuesday, will take him to the airport, Dad will fly via Atlanta because of the strike, wait over an hour, change planes, be met in San Francisco by Jean. (When I was there, he was rolling his eyes and couldn't talk.) I also realize it's just what

Jean wanted—not to have to go to Florida. So it all works out, and my plans—the two shifts of aides, the twenty-four hour sleep-in, the visiting boys, etc., etc.—were really superfluous. Good. I hope I remember next time.

More important, for this record, what happened to me in Florida. The mask in a way was a relief because it said what I couldn't say—"I can't take over." It was also disconcerting, as was being in a hospital, with the sick and the dying all around me. I felt diminished, anxious, a pretend invalid, torn between relief that I probably am not going to be old and senile and demanding, and fear that I will nevertheless end up like the bebagged, intravenoused characters I saw in the hall. (Will I be as demanding as Dad? As self-pitying? As disruptive? If indeed, he is disruptive— or I'm not just projecting.) As a footnote, my aunt Syrena, the brave one, turned out to be in the hospital in Palm Beach at the same time. She saw blood in her stools, was in the hospital by afternoon, had called my uncle Dan to come down, had "terrible tests," i.e., barium enema, etc., "came out clean, thank God" is now home, with Dan at her side. "How are you?" she asks when I call her. "Fine." "Still getting medication?" "Yes." "Why?" Again I tell her. "Oh," she says, and goes on to say, "How scared I was, you don't have to worry about me, I'm clean." Next minute Ellen calls to tell the sad tale of someone she knows who is "terminal," his wife's selfishness, his falling down, his not getting medicine fast enough, etc. Nuts. I know she's scared. But don't any of them *think?* . . . I hate the me in these pages these days, but I feel honor-bound.

To continue. The positives. It *was* a relief just to be there, to see that he was all right, and to realize it was not up to me any more.

Going into the apartment held no terrors. I routinely made up Mother's bed, lay down where she had died, patted the headboard with affection, found myself, truthfully, kissing the pillow, and settled back, feeling comfortable and happy to be there. At rest. A ghost dispatched. Many ghosts. Tilly, a mystery. Sixty-eight, Scarsdale-shiny, twice widowed, what she sees in Dad, etc. But she spoke of Mother, said he was a "perfect gentleman and more," and that it was good he had her, life goes on, and there was no pain in it at all.

But I got very tired as the days went on. The going back and forth to the hospital; the unending conversations, not eating, not resting, the endless tedious arrangements with agencies (my job), the long-distance calls, the explanations—whatever it was. I felt as though my strength was going out of me like sawdust from a doll, and my voice went. So the night I was so tired I couldn't sleep all night and my heart kept pounding, I decided to leave earlier. That decision made, I got up at three a.m., got to work on my as-it-turned-out useless lists, did more laundry, etc., and felt much less tired.

Saying goodbye to him was fraught, but I made it quick— all kinds of unsaid things in the air—and when I finally made my night plane I had one wish: I wanted a drink! Then finally Kennedy—and for the first time in many, many years I wanted the plane to land—and Vic met me, also for the first time, and that was over.

What did I find out?

I really wasn't pretending about not being able to take over. I don't have the stamina. My back goes, and my knee gets weak, among other things. Some of it, I still think, is emotional, but the fact is I do lead a fairly structured life. If I work, it's at home, for limited periods, and every once in a while I lie down, even if it's only for ten minutes. When I go out and walk around for any length of time, I lie down when I come back, again even if it's only for a short time. I have lots of quiet, too much sometimes. I eat when I feel like it. I don't know whether it's age, tension, the weak back, post-surgery, chemotherapy—or my head—but I was not the same woman who used to go tearing down to Hollywood every time Mother had an attack and commuted between hospital and apartment. (Actually I don't remember how I felt then. Maybe I was just as tired, but I didn't feel I had a right to admit it.)

I felt marked, set apart, because of the above, and I don't like it. I feel as if I took myself out of the mainstream—as I had to—and as if I must put myself back into it fast. Resume, where it's unspoken, not broadcast by mask or negation.

I found I got unreasonably angry at my father's helplessness and/or demands. In a way, it's reacting to past history; in a way, it's reacting to a feeling of being pushed; in a way, it's acknowledging what was unacknowledged, but it's overreaction, no question about it. Do I get upset by his behavior because I am afraid that is the way I will behave? (Aunt Syrena surprised me—I should have expected her to be much more stoic.) Am I afraid that I will be punished for my lack of sympathy by finding myself in exactly the same situation? (I should be horrified if Jan or Kathy reacted to me as I do to him—Vic reassures me that our relationship is different, and that my demands were different, but who knows? By Dad's lights he was a great father—and he still thinks of me as the "good" daughter.) Is there anger (as there may be in relation to my still-unresolved feeling about my mother) that we were picked out of turn, so to speak? That is, I was targeted ahead of him? It would be interesting, as I've said before, to see how I would have reacted and would react if I didn't have the cancer—but I'll never know.

(Such a dreary tale. Where fits in my walking up Madison Avenue in the clear fall sunshine on Friday, en route to Jetti Katz to have my blood checked, and my feeling so happy to be alive and well and home again that I could have burst with joy? Where fits my taking the train alongside the Hudson to meet Vic at Rhinebeck, delighting in the journey and the prospect of staying at the Beekman Arms overnight? Where fits my getting through a whole long Saturday, from Rhinebeck to Kingston, to Ancram to see the Fabers, arriving home near eleven, unpacking, doing mail, etc., without turning a hair except for wondering why social security should have called? Let's not go into *that* now.)

I don't know whether what I have been putting down is the belated beginning of wisdom, or the untimely relapse into infantilism. A little of both, I guess.

Or is it just that I am human?

I am reading galleys. I'll have to fix the acknowledgment of affection to Vic, the kids, "my father and my mother." It will come out in the spring, and I keep thinking that I have to provide for a possible message from the grave. (I mean it to be funny. Please.) In which case I would need a whole page of acknowledgments. I'll struggle with that tomorrow. It's still nice to have galleys.

Maybe what all the foregoing adds up to is that I haven't seen Mark for months. I have felt ill at ease. I shall be glad to see him tomorrow. (Will he find anything? I don't think so. But the medication, honestly, feels a little off. A projection, of course.)

Series 8

October 7. Mark is back, and the world is in place. In a way. Not so much to say because I say it here, and it's always the same somehow. Except that I got a start when he too cut the pills down to five. The white count, just on the borderline. "So it was so," I think, "I wasn't faking, I have to take care." Always a surprise.

I tell Mark that, of course, I don't live and move and breathe the thing—only in these pages when I'm writing—but now, a day after, I realize it isn't so. I do. Always the undercurrent. Because of the chemotherapy. Would I not be so aware if I didn't have to do something about it at least twice a week some weeks? A while ago walking to Knopf, I was thinking about—what? Death and dying. I don't know how it came into my mind, but I thought anew that it isn't dying that scares me, it's how. I know where it came from. I read an article about the immigrant Jews of New York while I was having lunch, and in it, Tillie Olson's story about her mother and father is mentioned. It was about her mother dying of cancer —I didn't remember that—and the part quoted tells of the old woman's body suffering. "Even dying is work, Mrs. Misfortune," says the old man, or something such. If only I could be guaranteed —my pain not to trouble anyone (preferably not me either)— and then I think of the time I am being given, and again, as if for the first time I realize, or try to, that actually I did have a recurrence, and that's why the chemotherapy, and my mind hurries to say, "No, it was just that they didn't see it the first time, then they did, and you know, it was really gone, better, taken care of." I think that my mother had ten years after her heart attack . . .

At Knopf it seems to me, again, that Gottlieb is frightened of me. At least, he treats me differently. Tentatively. No jokes. I know what it is—his mother, dead of cancer; his ambivalence about me (sometimes I'm his mother, sometimes I'm Maria, his young wife; never mind that he is the big publisher). And flatly I override it. I point out the acknowledgment—"my letter to the world," I say, "it really should be a lot longer." I don't say post-humous but that's in his head, and he says bluntly, "Why don't you write 'Thanks, world,'" and we go on to the next subject.

Small world department: On Gottlieb's desk, ready to come out, is a first book by Kathy's once great and good friend, Mark Helprin. Ten years ago I read his English class papers and was jealous of what a good writer he was. Now I am handing in the galleys of my fourth novel—and he is hailed on the jacket "as a born teller of tales." I read the book later, make up a note to him, telling him the turn our fates have taken, and feel the note would be incomplete unless I tell him about the cancer. Why? Because as a writer, he would relish the double switch. Who knows? It doesn't seem to make sense to write him unless I do—it would feel like masquerading—but I won't, of course.

Social security calls. I am eligible for some disability. I don't know how to react. Glad, because they think I can't work? Sad? Pleased at being able to stand on my own a little? (I have been feeling very, very dependent these last long months.) Pleased that I was matter of fact and sensible for once? I thank the woman at the other end of the telephone, and she says, "Just take care of yourself, and stay well, hear?" What did Mark say on the medical form? (It is not possible to win. Not ever.)

As I left Knopf, I passed Jan's office, got her, had coffee in the little park next door. Lovely. Light and shade. Life.

I feel very incompetent at expressing what I feel. I am obliged to anecdote, but what I feel in need of is a philosophy. It'll come maybe.

I woke up at six thirty this morning with a start. A feeling of being trapped. Terrifying. Like going under anesthesia, swept up in a process over which you have no control. I am in a prison from which there is no exit.

I try to reason myself out of it. In reality I feel fine. A little puffy, I think—my fingers are on the largish side (I measure by where my big ring goes, it varies from third to second—of course my regular rings, wedding ring, diamond, don't go on at all), my nose a bit spread, some of my dis-ease may be a little more edema than usual (possibly because it is suddenly warm again), a sort of pre-menstrual feeling. Where soma, where psyche?

Is it because I *have* nothing to worry about? Nothing extra, that is. Or because I have nothing much to do with this day that is to come? No, actually I do have plans, so it's not that. But the world seems flat. I'm not interested in anything much (now, at seven o'clock—or at least, trying to re-create how I felt a few hours ago).

If I were really at work—absorbed—it would be better.

I muddle through the morning. Read the *Times.* Wait for the man to fix the blinds. Arrange where to meet Hattie. Ponder whether to swim now, or later. (I should be doing something for people, volunteering, something, shouldn't I? But that's evasive—right now. When I can't do anything else, then I will—selfishly.) And then my father calls—seven thirty in California. Or rather, Jean does first. The trip was good, he's fine, he has told her she is not to be tied down but to come and go as she has to, she can get a visiting nurse for a couple of hours because the doctor sent a letter along. I marvel, and she says, "Don't think I haven't been working on it. One day I decided not to call Florida, I just did my lesson and closed the books and decided I had done and thought and agonized all I could, now it was out of my hands." After which, she says, the doctor decided he could come to California, the plans were made, and she was told what she had to do. Which was what she wanted to do all along.

Then my father gets on. Calm. Content. No problem traveling even though the trip took seven hours. "I'm happy to be here. Take care of yourself."

I feel chastened, tearful, somehow out of the depression. Again, what can I learn from this? I write a note to them to try to tell them how pleased I was to hear them both sound the way they did, but I really can't make it clear. I overreact. I am a doddering Hamlet convinced that by cursed spite, my role is to make everything right (always was, that's no different), but I don't *want* to do it, I resent the obligation—and really, all along, I'm the one that does it to me, no one else, and if I just let things roll, everyone, especially and including me, would be better off.

Again—my mantra should be "Let go," "Let go"—don't anticipate, don't worry about what may be, just live in the here and now, be grateful for what is.

Let time stand still. I don't ask to be better (better how?). Just let my body be as it is. Do I really want time to stand still? There are days that seem to be death-takes-a-holiday days, and they're very disconcerting . . . I see that in the space of a para-

graph I am back to trying to control. Making bargains. (Avoiding working by working on this—aha, you can't fool me, this is
only an illusion of work. Cheaper than psychiatry though—reality
is reality. And, mirabile dictu, as usual, I've typed myself out of a
corner. Welcome, O life! Peace. Om. Down. What is, is. Into thy
hands. Somewhere inside me is a layer of serenity, let me reach
into it. Or is the layer outside me, and do I reach out to it? It is
very hard to refrain from faith even when you fear you are making
it up yourself.

October 11. A Day in the Life. Halfway through the morning the mail brought a packet from Senator Kennedy. A Xerox of
a letter from the National Cancer Institute obviously in response
to a Xerox of my letter to him because Rauscher, the director,
writes to Kennedy(!) that he is sorry his "correspondent is a cancer patient" but "is pleased to know she is responding well to
chemotherapy." On the heroin question, he writes "heroin is indeed an effective analgesic" but the drug is a Schedule 1 drug, and
would create "difficulties" because of the risk of it getting into the
hands of "hard" users is great. Therefore, the NCI "has never conducted studies with heroin and has no plans to do so." He enclosed
a good deal of material about cancer, chemotherapy and an article
on the relief of pain.

I am overwhelmed at first. I read the article—by a William
Derrick, M.D., of the Anderson Hospital and Tumor Institute—
and, alas, find not so much methods of relief, as the various forms
cancer pain can take which I had never thought of—broken bones,
among them. The palliatives, little though I think I have read, are
all familiar to me. Then I try to decide whether I should read the
literature, "Drugs vs. Cancer," "Treating Cancer," "Science and
Cancer." I recognize Alkeran and find out what it does—maybe—
guess about my other drugs; learn, in toto, very little, except that
(a) it is all uncertain and (b) nobody really knows but (c) great
progress has been made and everyone is hopeful, of what they

really don't quite know. Result: I am uneasy (all that reality creeping up on me) but not surprised.

I decide, however, to write one more letter to Kennedy, thanking him, and pointing out that not doing something because addicts (who already seem pretty well supplied to me) may possibly latch on to it seems peculiar, if not appalling.

The morning shot, I go to spend an afternoon with my friend Janet, who, as she says, is "also afflicted." I decide we will not talk about "it." At lunch she describes her brother's current coronary bypass surgery, and inevitably we get onto the subject of how long life is worth living, what measures one should take, etc., etc. Her brother, still recovering, questions whether he should have gone through the trauma of surgery. "I've had a good life, I'm sixty," etc. Her reply: "If God had wanted you, he would have taken you, but obviously he's not ready for either of us yet. He's just nudged us." More peripheral talk, and she asks me how long I am going to be on chemotherapy (she isn't). I explain that I don't know, and don't ask, because who knows? "You're the question asker," I say. "Obviously, that's why I asked you." "Well," I say, "I wasn't going to tell you, but . . ." and I tell her of the Kennedy packet, and how it also ends up with the usual uncertainties. Which I find encouraging. So she asks me if I have seen the book on breast cancer which was reviewed in the *Times.* I say I've seen the review which, it turns out, is all she saw. She reports that the statistics terrified her—and some of her friends, who have also had mastectomies. I tell her I thought they were encouraging—after all, fifty-fifty. And then we talk about how people cope—writing the book was obviously one way of Mrs. Kushner's coping—she talks about herself —she tried to join the group that visits mastectomy patients as soon as she was out of the hospital but was refused. Five years, they said, "and I realize now it isn't so much the survival part, but that your motives are very mixed in the beginning." I mention that this journal is one way I cope, and she asks me what I put in it.

I tell her—and decide to give an example of the essentially unsayable—i.e., the thinking of my having a mastectomy preced-

ing my making love, only I change the thought to colostomy when
I verbalize it to Janet. She nods. Then she says that her husband, a
doctor, who had, I know, made her stop dressing in bathrooms and
hiding behind towels, "Hasn't yet put his hand on the scar." "Have
you?" I ask, and then go on to say Vic has flinched at my stitch, it's
just one of those things, probably a good way of avoiding seeing
that we are different. "You haven't got what I have, the mutilation," she says, my pretty, delicate, silver-blond friend. I laugh, and
tell her how one of my fantasies is that that would be all right, it's
outside of one. No, it isn't, she says. "Should we be talking like this
over our nice lunch?" I say, knowing the answer. "Why not?" she
says, and she's right. It's a heady feeling, walking into the forbidden, in a way. There is really no one else to whom we can talk
quite like this, we realize. Then I ask her if it's always with her. I
say I'm worried that my journal gives the idea that it's all I ever
think of, and she interrupts to say, "But that's all I ever think of.
No matter what I do, it's always in the background." So then I
mention the pain correspondence, and she says, "That doesn't
worry me at all. I just know that something would be done. Jack
wouldn't let me suffer, nor would anyone else. And no one would
let you suffer either." So I tell her of the talk I had with Kathy
after my first surgery, when she said they had looked at the bottle
of sleeping pills Phil had prescribed, thought about it, and left it
there, and I told her it was right, I wouldn't do anything (I
thought). She said they had decided (she, Jan, and Vic) that anything like that would be a mutual decision. Janet frowns. "A terrible responsibility," she says. "Words," I say, and I tell her Kathy
is pregnant and my first reaction, "I'll see the baby." Important to
Kathy, I say, and she asks if I thought it was a good idea to have
conversations like that with Kathy. Well, I tell her, they're really
quite unreal—I do it for these pages, so I become my alter ego.
"The games people play," says Janet, and we go off to the Islamic
exhibition.

   We look and enjoy it and at the very end Janet says what she
said after we saw the Scythian gold, "All of this makes me feel

how unimportant we all are, how anything that happens to us is meaningless." Mountains do it for her too, she says, and I tell her of my feeling before I was sick about putting the Milky Way in a hospital room, a sense of immensities should put things in perspective, but when I was waiting for a scan and saw the pictures of a galaxy in *Scientific American,* I was frightened. "Oh," says Janet, "it terrifies me." So, torn between time and space, we make our way out and are caught up by a pair of wooden Han figures from the second century B.C. that neither of us had ever seen in the Chinese rooms. Breathtaking. Humanizing. And we both feel good.

And so we leave the museum, I to go to Jetti Katz for a blood test, she down the block toward home. "Come back for a drink," she says, and surprisingly I do. We drink, and we talk some more. This time of how essentially *little* we share with our husbands of this kind of thing, because we know it would hurt them. Besides, we agree, women are better able to face feelings, or voice them, anyway. Or maybe it's just that we have more time, and so we are back to our old topic of guilt—both of us, for not working. Only she says she thinks she has it licked. "I'm glad to be making my own schedule," she says. "Besides," I add, "the world will go on whether I sit at my typewriter or not." Janet agrees, and both of us, with the same impulse, change the subject. *Ragtime vs. Waiting for Mr. Goodbar,* it is.

Next day—today—I go to a woman I have found in the Yellow Pages to have my face waxed. She turns out to be European, blond, fragile—and the waxing turns out to be very painful and unpleasant. As I sit in her oddly furnished apartment (it almost looks as if she had just been divorced and her husband took half the furniture), I feel as though it is just too much. The wax hardening on my cheeks, all this to be done over and over again—too much. Then I tell myself how lucky I am to be able to have it done, this should be the least, etc., etc. (I remember the pamphlet on drug therapy that says after a while the drugs don't work—but how will they know when that is, how do they know how the drugs are working on me anyway, there isn't anything it's reducing, I don't think.) She comes in to pull the second strip of wax off and I see the blue-black numbers on her arm. Bastards. They even put the line through the number 7. She is very kind, apologetic for hurting, says it will be easier next time, makes up some bleach for me to use in between times. I want to say something to her, but I can't find any words.

Walking home I think of Sissman's remark that any long-term regimen is "deadening to the spirit." Is that what this is? A plateau, I trust. It had better be.

October 12. Pathetic fallacy in action—rain since yesterday, the country dreary, as was I. Ellen called as soon as I got there—this time she not only gave me her symptoms but, as if tuned into me, a story about W. S. (terminal), and an exclamation about how "stupid he was, he should have taken pills weeks ago, and spared Abby all this trouble, he's crazy now, eighty pounds," etc., etc. Trying to change the subject, mentioned another friend—"Oh, she's dead," said Ellen. "Your beautiful friend!" I said. "Not so beautiful when they got through giving her chemotherapy." How did she die? "Well, they said her sickness, but I think she must have taken something. The way Walter should have." End of conversation.

I can't tell her not to—it would put me in her power somehow—and I don't know if it's intentional, it started with, "Donald says you look so well," but I think it's in me. I feel as though I am having my back forced to the wall.

So I wake up with it in the morning—terrified somehow—and later in the morning, I am amused because Vic is having the grandchildren recite Shakespeare. "To be or not to be," they shout, over and over again, and then, "Tomorrow and tomorrow and tomorrow," and for a while it becomes funny. Then I read Rachel MacKenzie's *Risk,* about heart surgery (research for the possible book), and become very emotional inside, because all surgery somehow has common elements, and it brings back something suppressed. As I close the book, Vic looks at me and says, "Are you all right?" and I begin to cry. First, or almost first time. Dilemma— to tell or not to tell. I decide to tell him. "I'm scared," I say. "Why?" "I don't know," and I really don't, unless it's the accumulation of the past week, the plateau, or maybe—new thought—I am secure enough not to be suppressing. At any rate, I say a little of what I was thinking, and point out that I know sharing this is divisive, but not sharing is also separating, and I don't know the answer. "Say whatever you feel," he says, but I see that now *he* feels trapped. "There isn't anything you can say, is there?" I say, and he nods his head. Helpless. Then he suggests I should see my psychiatrist friend Michael, who deals with his own heart condition by denying it (denying it? having a really marvelous, busy time— coincidence, I suppose—also, he has his work, his two presidencies, Erica, etc., etc. I know that part of my problem is that I have nothing I *have* to do), and I say I don't need a psychiatrist, this is reality, and I cope pretty well, and sometimes I am just not going to cope, I am only human.

Actually I didn't say the above, only that I don't need psychiatry (do I? I really don't think so). And it is hard for me to re-create the feeling, because right now I don't have it—partly because I spoke, partly because I got busy, partly because the sun is now out.

Roy just called to speak to Vic. "I'm so glad you're feeling better," he says.

"Better? But I've always been fine," I said. "Maybe my back . . ."

"No," he says, "I'm just glad you're okay."

He means well, but he makes me queasy. Fact.

.   .   .

Saw old friends last night. Haven't seen them for more than a year. They do not comment upon my weight, do not ask what has happened to me during the last year (not anything, not even the book), and mirabile dictu, I say nothing (although I am very aware of last year's long skirt not closing). And I feel like me again. Vic, however, is silent on the way home, and I begin to feel a little guilty. Please let me keep my mouth shut henceforth because in some ways, I really sound worse than I feel.

October 13. Off the plateau, I think—this time. It seemed to peak last night after a good day with the family—much laughter and busyness—when Vic stayed up late watching the late, late something (rejection, thought I, naturally), and I tried to sleep, and couldn't. Some anger ensued and I decided to take one 2 mg. Valium "to break the cycle" (first since the height of the backache —it's against my religion to use pills to change my emotions). Then a realization that I, not he, was rejecting by withdrawing into my hurt shell, etc. All thereafter well, and I slept, and woke up feeling qualitatively different. (Sun was shining again; too.)

To Mark, and cycle was completed. Told him about the plateau and/or depression, and gave him the Kennedy material. (When he offered to give it back to me, I realized I didn't want it. Who needs booklets labeled "Cancer" around the house? Not me.) As usual, dear Mark, you speak to my condition. First he suggested that some malaise may be hormonal, chemical, whatever. Perfectly true (I had that sense last week). Also, we agreed that I have had ups and downs before, everyone does, only now I label them. And then, later, I think he put his finger on what I have been going through these past weeks—I have been puzzled about the present as much as the future. "I'm not a prophet," he said, and I finished the thought for him (as usual, interrupting before a thought is completed). I'm okay now, but I act as if I'm not, or try to order my thoughts as if I were dying when, in fact, I'm living. All the emphasis on death and dying that is in the culture, to be sure, as well as in me, only compounds my problem. I'm overanticipating. And Mark's analogy of death as the last quotation mark was very exciting—what is in the quotation before is living, not dying, as long as you're alive, etc., etc. (Christ, the banalities of these discoveries, as they are discovered over and over and over again!) And he told me the story of the eighty-eight-year-old woman who just wants to be well enough for "two weeks in Florida." My banner for the day—two weeks in Florida. Whatever —I'm okay.

So I drove home, consciously enjoying the process of driving itself, zipping to the Deegan, swerving on the Willis, speeding up on the East River Drive; tried to go swimming—no soap, pool was filthy, every fly has its ointment, right?—bicycled two miles on the stationary cycle instead; went marketing, had lunch (consciously enjoying it), and absolutely conked out for two hours. I was exhausted by whatever went before, no question about it, and I needed to lie down to complete my recovery from it.

Later I tried to explain what I had talked about with Mark to Jan. One of the few times, but she was over yesterday and when we went for a walk, I said something about how I was feeling. Purposely. "But you are more conscious of mortality than people your age," she said, "you can't avoid it, don't denigrate your thoughts, you are dying in a way." And I really felt she had it wrong—she is too young to understand that what I am talking about, what we were talking about—is not denial, but a way of life. What is, is. For some reason I think of Simone Weil saying she had to love her suffering, not because it was good or enobling, but because it was. I propose to love my *non*-suffering. After all, everything is a leap of faith; even, for me, turning on a light. I don't know how it is accomplished.

From *The World of Zen:*

God—if I may borrow the word—the universe, and man are one indissoluble existence, one total whole. Only This—capital This—is. Anything and everything that appears to us as an individual entity or phenomenon, whether it be a planet or an atom, a mouse or a man, is but a temporary manifestation of This in form; every activity that takes place, whether it be birth or death, loving or eating breakfast, is but a temporary manifestation of This in activity. When we look at things this way, naturally we cannot believe that each individual person has been endowed with a special and individual soul or self. Each one of us is but a cell, as it were, in the body of the Great Self, a cell that comes into being, performs its functions, and passes away, transformed into another manifestation. Though we have temporary individuality, that temporary, limited individuality is not either a true self or our true self. Our true self is the Great Self; our true body is the Body of Reality . . .

Reading the line about the cell, I choke. For a moment I have what apparently is defined as a nonintellectual illumination. But by the time I sit down to type the passage, the illumination has passed. Still, for the moment, it was. Part of the problem was that while I was typing, the book kept slipping and closing. A parable—koan, if you will—of the whole situation. Another koan —as I close the book it opens to a charcoal drawing of a doctor's spoon. The characters, translated, are said to read: "Whether for life or whether for death depends on what's in the spoon." Ponder.

October 21. Haven't written in nearly a week, I think. Sign of serenity? Not really. I've been busier, and my thinking has moved a cog—away from cancer, in a sense; right there, in another.

I have been reading old files, and suddenly—about a half hour ago I got into a panic. I feel deserted, alone (phone hasn't rung!), cut off, existential. I decided at eleven o'clock that I would spend the next hour putting my life to rights. Nice idea. Where to begin? First thought was to list people I really want to see, to have in my life. Next I looked at my bookshelves. But finally, I settled here—to see if I can figure out what is happening.

First thing that comes to mind is that living from day to day has caught up with me. The *Atlantic* has a piece on Hiroshima by Robert Lifton in which he tells of how some of the hurt survivors have made a way of life out of their radiation exposure—the trips to the doctors, the talking, the questioning. They are Witnesses, and it is important, I suppose, like remembering the Holocaust. On the other hand, those who are participating in the rebirth of Hiroshima resent them, they wish only to look forward. Typing this I see that the latter miss the point. The survivors have never been sure they had anything to look forward to—not even children because of the worry about genetic damage. But it's been a long time . . . Anyway what rings a bell for me is the way of life in doctoring. Mondays to the Bronx, Fridays to the lab, it gives an illusion of activity, the way going to a psychiatrist when I wasn't working expanded to take up the whole day. That's point 1 —how to absorb the treatments. (I'm fudging here—it's only the Mondays, the lab visits don't mean a thing, I do absorb them. The point is to see what I do with the time between.)

I have also been escaping—the weekends—I noticed that even driving back from Cambridge in the rain and the fog, I had my airplane-landing syndrome for a minute, I didn't want to arrive, I was happy just to be in limbo.

I got my disability check and wanted to give it to Vic. Shades of the time I surprised him by paying the obstetrician in advance for Jan! He wouldn't take it. I should have known. *He* pays the bills. Well, I'm glad, even though subliminally they're there—in case. It still makes me feel better—in a way. In another way, it troubles me because it is more of the day to day business. Still I read a way out. If I earn anything I am to notify them, and the checks stop for that period. As usual I have made of the flat-out ordinary event an internal moral battle.

Which brings me to Zen. I have been reading, but—and maybe this is the point of it—as soon as I get an inkling I get hit on the head. To wit: He who truly attains awakening knows that deliverance is to be found right where he is . . . to handle Reality itself, and by handling it to awaken to the state of Reality . . . every act from morning to evening is religion . . .

What does this mean? Aside from putting down your buckets where you are? That accepting what is is itself a religion. Well, I can go on about that, but the trouble is that I cannot accept all the anecdotes that are given as explanation. For example: A monk comes to see the Abbot of Nansen and encounters a woodcutter. He asks if the Abbot is at home and the woodcutter lifts up his axe and holds it over the monk's head threateningly, saying, "It is very sharp." The monk flees, later learns the woodcutter was Nansen. Same thing throughout; ask a question, you get a nonsense reply, or a bop. Why? Salvation so far does not lie in Zen.

Okay. To go on with this stream of consciousness. I feel cramped (I almost feel it physically as I write, my skin stretched, my bones like a cage). I know that I have been dawdling away my days, and I blame myself for it, but I wonder, as I am plowing through these pages trying to find out why, whether that door at the end of the shortened corridor isn't psychologically blocking my way. (It begins to feel right as I write this.) I don't register for courses, start anything . . . no, that's not the reason. The latter I don't do because I know it would be a distraction, not my real work.

There are several, conflicting blocks, I see. On the one hand, I am suddenly extremely interested in TM, Zen, philosophy, etc. —obviously—I need to make sense of life, not only because of the cancer, I always groped. That has just made it a little more urgent. But I keep putting off any serious exploration for "when I'll need it," i.e., in some near, but not comprehensible, future. The problem is will I be in a condition to do it when I need it?

This too—a journal of a plague year—it is a framework for something I can do when I know how it will end, or that it is ending.

So the two matters that interest me most now—the search and the theme—I put aside because I don't feel I am ready yet—or that the time is appropriate. To say that it is, is to admit a defeat, or at least an ending.

But the other—living—doesn't interest me as much. (Interesting word—"living"—as opposed to—what?) And since I can only work now on what interests me—what drives me—or so it seems.

All the while I've been typing this I have been glancing up to see the title *The Denial of Death,* the book Becker finished just before he died . . .

Have I been blocked because I have thought that whatever I do has to be a final statement? Afraid to begin because the sea, as always, looks limitless? I keep seeing Mark's analogy of the quotation mark—maybe I have to incorporate into my work too the idea that "———— is ordinary, daily, just work until the time for" arrives. Which isn't now.

Too much pigeon-holing. Why don't I do a little of everything and try to bring as much richness into my days as they will hold? Because that's how it should be always.

October 28. Good sign. Days without journal. Days without ego? (I reread some of Anaïs Nin's diaries and began to understand what appears to be so much overweening self-importance. If you're writing about yourself, you do get terribly one-track. And if it's a journal, not a piece of fiction, it tends to be flat-out. She complains that the journal is keeping her from "real" writing.)

We went back to Sarasota for the weekend. Another milestone (like getting back the fur coat I didn't have fixed because the furrier said it would "last forever" when I took it in to be stored over the summer). Beautiful, untouched, preserved in amber, Sarasota.

I walk in the door and say to myself, "Laude." (Earlier in the week I heard the "Laude" from the Bernstein mass sung as an encore and I wept. For joy.) Then I swim in the gulf and, floating in the sea, a pelican companionably at my left, and the gulls swooping, I think of how each time I am grateful to be here and wonder whether I will come back, and then I do come back, and "laude, laude." Then I wonder. Is being grateful itself neurotic? Shouldn't I be taking it for granted I will be back? In the sea? Writing the question I know the answer. No, I shouldn't be taking it for granted, not now, and not before, and not in the future. Being aware is one of the pluses. Why dilute it?

It is an easy four days. I barely think about it (it? cancer? my four-letter word), except to think I'm not thinking about it. And then we go home and when the plane lands, I'm not even sorry. I even have a surge of joy as we go over the Fifty-ninth Street bridge and I see the lights of the city. What is more, I have planned a dinner party for the day after I get back with only the slightest question whether I will be there for it. After all, four days!

Oddities of people:

I call my aunt Syrena who had a polyp removed in Palm Beach. She is greatly relieved to be "all clean," according to the biopsy. Complains about the hospital, the enemas, etc. (my non-complaining aunt). Next breath she asks how I am. "Fine," I say. "You always say that," she protests, "are you *really* fine?"

I call my father, back in Hollywood, Florida. He is well. "How are you?" he asks. "All better?" "Yes." "Did your treatments do you good?" I assure him yes. I guess he doesn't understand, but why should he? Essentially no one else does, including me.

Then my friend Elmer calls. My good old friend of forty years, and more. He talks and talks and then says—after he has asked me how I am—that he has bad news. His oldest friend—an acquaintance of mine—is dying of cancer of the liver. I say I am sorry. He says he is getting chemotherapy but another friend, a doctor, says he shouldn't be because it only prolongs things and "makes you feel lousy." He also says it is going very fast. I make the proper noises and suddenly I change my mind. "Chemotherapy doesn't make me feel lousy," I say. Also, "If he is really dying, it's a good thing it's going fast." "I guess so," says Elmer miserably. It is apparent he really doesn't connect me and Joe—and I guess he's right. It *is* different. But I am expecting my six guests momentarily. I am all dressed up in brown, but for a minute I feel like a white sepulcher. It passes when the bell rings, but all evening long I am aware of a little undercurrent in me. As if I am play-acting.

In the morning I wake up with a quotation—"When in disgrace with fortune and men's eyes . . ." I think about it for a while and then wonder. Am I in disgrace with fortune? It is a childhood quotation and I think I thought it had to do somehow with Shakespeare losing his money. But I realize it's not that—it's fortune banishing him. Has fortune banished me? I don't think so at all, but maybe I'm fooling myself. I get nowhere with it, only a faint sense of unease. So I spend the day running—happily. I swim, I do two miles on the bike, I market, I walk to meet Jane in the park and have coffee, I walk back, I collapse, I cook for Kathy, I do everything except what I should do—get to work.

Still, why work? Gottlieb yesterday said Joseph Heller spent twelve years happily "having written *Catch-22*." Ah, but I haven't written *Catch-22*. Does that make a difference? To me, yes. Even if I had, it would still matter. But there is a time for filling up, that I know (do I have the time? If I don't, it doesn't matter anyway because the writing is for me, I don't fancy myself giving the world anything). And also, there is a time for enjoying, and if today I enjoy running . . . what makes Sammy run? Fear. I wrote the last on a slip of paper yesterday, but it doesn't apply right now. It's smart-alecky. I just hope the spirit moves soon. I do enjoy words coming out of my fingers.

October 30. Woke up this morning remembering I had forgotten some things. The trouble with *not* thinking about it all the time, and taking notes, is that nuances get overlooked. To wit:

• Swimming at Sarasota (somehow all my epiphanies are connected with water—water always seems to signify rebirth—*if* I believed in such things, I would ascribe it to my Piscean nature and my adopted god, Ea, the Babylonian, who turns out to be the

sign of the fish—but enough of this, I'm writing now, not journal-
ing), I feel my limbs moving strongly, think of the elation I felt
the first time I felt myself moving in this same water six weeks
after my first surgery, quickly summarize operations and recoveries,
anticipate my dying, decide I won't die of cancer, but of a heart
attack (in my sleep naturally—family tradition), willed by me
(control, control), and swim happily on, all of this taking perhaps
thirty seconds, a minute at the most. Why not? I think to myself.
I can just as well believe that as anything else. That night, naturally, I feel twinges in my chest (after a heavy dinner and wine, to
be sure, and the fatigue of sun and swimming and riding the stationary bike in the sauna room). "Oh, no," I say to myself, "too
soon, that's not part of the agreement, I'm not ready!" A day or
two later, I get up after lying down reading a small-print mystery
and find myself dizzy, reeling across the room. Shaken, I say again,
"Not yet, not yet," and remember that about a month ago, lying
down, in the dark, the bedroom began to turn. Lasted a minute or
so. Indigestion, circulation problem, post-coitus (both instances
happened to be), who knows? I sat in a chair at poolside after the
dizzy spell and watched the top of my bathing suit rise and fall,
trying to figure whether my heart was palpitating too fast. Was it
really or was I paying attention? I couldn't decide. BUT—I began
to think that maybe the price for *time* is worth paying. I couldn't
decide whether I was pleased at the hurried heartbeats or not—had
the mental picture of pushing my shoulder against the door where
two demons were trying to get in. The trick is to allow only one—
the *right* one—to slip by *when* I am ready, and not before. Primitive, infantile, manipulative—still, the game gives me amusement
—*and* a sense of power.

   • I watch the condominium dwellers. Two or three years ago
they looked different. Now the same people seem calmer, tanner,
somehow more at peace. I ask one of the women about it, and she
agrees. "We've all learned we all have problems, we've come to
accept each other." They also seemed to have found their respective
ways of life—the women more seeking than the men, the men

somehow more companionable. (The big thing on the bulletin board now is TM and yoga—for the women.) I feel totally alien to them. Always did. I can't picture myself their age, although I probably am, or living their life. But more than that I can't picture us growing old, or even older, together. We exist. Period.

• I watch myself—no, watch is inaccurate—now and then I catch a glimpse of myself in a mirror and I don't recognize my body. My heavier arms, my pot belly, my thickened waist, my fuzzy cheeks. It bothers me very little though, because I assume no one else really notices except me—that it's as though my shadow has become broader but the real me is still slim. Even though one of the condominium ladies says, seeing me in my bathing suit (same one as last year though): "You look marvelous! You're heavier!" Indeed.

• Kathy comes to visit, wearing one of my too-small skirts, which takes the place of one of her now too-small skirts. She has a small pot belly, her arms are fatter, her waist is thickened. She pats her belly; I pat mine. I make her dinner, and as we eat, hungrily, we compare the vitamins we are taking which presumably are making us so hungry. She speaks of being dizzy, having had a scary dizzy spell; I mention mine. Then it strikes me that something crazy is happening, and I hope she doesn't realize it. We are comparing symptoms! But she is carrying life—I suppose you would have to say I am carrying death. Well, you might have to say it, but it is a bit overdramatized. I am carrying hormones, life-giving, hopefully, hormones; I am giving life to myself. (Well, I got out of that one pretty well, didn't I?)

• A "friend" has done something very hurtful. It involves Vic even more than me, and so hurt I cannot keep it to myself. I tell him. He is outraged, insists I face my anger for once. I do. If not now, when? Anger turned inward, as well I know, is corrosive. I promise to do something about it, but before I can, he does. Result: end of friendship. I brood. It happened weeks ago. Finally I decide she may not have meant to hurt, maybe she was trying to protect me, however mistaken and ill-advised it was. I ask Vic if we can't somehow patch it up (really she should have apologized, but she won't, I know; can't, that's what she is like). Life is too short. But he is still too outraged. Problem—stated at its most succinct: is life too short to be taking shit, or is life too short to mind it? I have a sad feeling I am more comfortable with the latter out.

• Change of pace—can't end on that note—Kim, talking to Kathy about names for her offspring, suggests Victoria, Elizabeth, Mary (suffering surfeit of English royalty obviously). Kathy says they're nice names but points out they're "not Jewish." Kim has no idea there are "Jewish" names. Kathy explains. "But," asks Kim, "how do you know the baby is going to be Jewish?"

• From the current column in the *Atlantic* I surmise my pen friend Sissman is forty-five. That means he got Hodgkin's in his midthirties. I also have gleaned from other columns that he was married, for the second time, around the same period. He's had a time, hasn't he? For some reason I feel awe. So young, and to have handled it all with such grace. I think, How do I know? Because he writes gracefully? Because grass is always greener? No. Because I can sense it.

November 1. Kathy also seems to have picked up on our comparing of symptoms, only she put it differently. Speaking of the sense of being "invaded"—of having no control over her body any more—she said, "It's the way you must feel." I took a deep breath inside, then tried to re-create the way I had changed it in my thoughts, the chemotherapy being the active agent, not cells. I would hate her to have *that* connection. I also did something I haven't before—built up how very well I am, cancer-free, etc.— mostly by quoting Dr. Bulkin and then Mark too. "I'm not a prophet, but," etc. Then she picked up Mark's statement about my being "unique" (post-surgery) and how "remarkably" I am doing with chemotherapy, and I see that she has worked out a whole routine for handling it. Good. (I had told her of my Kennedy corre-

spondence, and the uncertainties—which I find comforting—like
the story yesterday about the Russian WHO doctor who says four
out of ten cancer victims in the Soviet Union have had five-year
cures—*any* statistic pleases me.) It seems to me some of the emotion and tension have gone out of the subject for us.

Footnote: Kathy reported that each person at a recent conference she attended was told to turn to his neighbor and say something about himself. All she could think of was, "I am pregnant,"
so, apologetically and explaining, she said it. It's all that's on her
mind. Me too. Encountering someone I haven't seen in a while, or
writing someone, my first, mental answer is always, "I have (had)
cancer." I don't always say it, try not to, but then I feel that I am
somehow cheating by omission. Is it the most important thing
about me right now? At the moment it seems highly unreal. Someone else maybe, not me.

November 2. I see my wax lady again (three weeks—in between I have put on a bleach she gave me and except for a gold
fuzz I am all right). This time (as she says) she is more "heroic."
Do I have children? she asks me. When I say yes, she asks what
they do, in order to tell me about hers—one at Barnard, one at
Yale, trying to get into medical school. "You did well," I say,
thinking of that damned tattoo on her arm. "Oh, yes," she says,
"but my husband is American." The thought is never out of her
mind, either, I'm sure.

On Sunday I see Lester, my son-in-law, in the living room
and for the moment he reminds me of my grandfather, or rather,
the picture I have seen of my grandfather. "He was the hand-
somest man around," I tell Lester. "He was twenty-nine or thirty
when he died. Pneumonia." Lester is taken aback. "I never knew
about him," he said. Then he tells how his father "almost died" as
a child; I counter with Vic's pneumonia at twenty. "We don't

know anything about death," Lester says. "We grow up ignorant until we're thirty, thirty-five, and then it hits us." He's thirty-five . . . (So young. I never quite realized it. Father of a ten-year-old. But then so was Vic. I was trying to place myself in age the other day. Thirty-six when we moved to Pleasantville. Did I feel young? A child dependent on my parents? Shy about making friends? Maybe the latter—but not because of age. I felt as old as I do now. And as experienced. More so. Then I didn't realize how much was beyond my emotional grasp. No, they won't miss me that way. They're grown up, and must feel so inside. But how about Kathy's touching collapse into tears Saturday morning and her joy at being put to bed with hot milk? First trimester pregnancy regression. I love that last. Label, and all the pulls and passions are trivialized. Anyway, I guess I am grown up too. I remember my sorority housemother, Mrs. Abendschein, bigoted, loving, neurotic. Mrs. Evening Glow. Whistler's Mother, literally as to costume, at seventy plus—was that all she was? She seemed centuries old— when I asked her why I felt no different on my eighteenth birthday than I had felt the day before, she said, "Thee will find that inside, thee is always the same age." The same anything. Regardless.)

Lester and I took a long walk, following the kids into the woods. Then we sat on the hill for a long time and talked. Like the old days. First time since . . . and as I write I realize it's not true at all. We walked together in Nantucket and talked . . . still, for some reason, it had a different feeling this time. In Nantucket, we were proving something—that I was okay (the residue of the back?), and wasn't it great I could keep up! Now it was normal. Unself-conscious until this very moment when I am suddenly attaching meaning. Self-conscious or aware? There *is* a difference, isn't there?

This journal is so dull—for which God be thanked, no?

.   .

Three miles on the bike yesterday, some swimming, walking to Fifth Avenue and Fifty-seventh, and back, and marketing, and walking again last night. Did I get tired? Absolutely! The exercise has an underlay. Not so much keeping myself as preparing . . . I think. Plus pleasure in seeing my body respond with more vigor each time. But self-conscious, oh, very self-conscious. Even to being aware that unlike the other women I cannot be casual about the towel around my abdomen. On the other hand, why not?

November 5. After nearly three years (must be, it certainly preceded the surgery) I grow tired of looking at my damaged big toe. Yesterday the nail had a large black ridge across it; last week there was a small black spot. Periodically I have thought it was renewing itself; a nail isn't much to bother with, and besides, under the circumstances . . . But I decide I apparently am going to outlive the nail so I go to see a Doctor McCarthy, who may sound Irish but acts Jewish. He calls me Violet right off, asks me if I am on any medication, and when I tell him what, he counters with the wild story of his sister, aged twenty-nine, who kept putting off her hysterectomy as her Pap smears got worse and worse ("plus two, plus three, finally four, finish!"). "Malignant?" I say. "Yes," he says, "but she got married a couple of months later anyway and since she already had a child from her first marriage, they didn't want one, so it worked out fine. Trouble is she has so much trouble with her weight, she's gained fifteen pounds already, no spaghetti, everything plain in her cooking, and still, she's built, you know what I mean!" He also confides in me that she thought she wouldn't have to use Tampax any more but she still bleeds. And is getting chemotherapy. "For a year only, they said, then she stops." Sister McCarthy boggles my mind. Her age, her marriage, her apparent ebullience, her symptoms. I hope Doctor McCarthy sees she gets good care (he was recommended by Rifkin, but her surgery was not at Rifkin's hospital so I don't know); he won't give me pills for what he says is a fungus caused by blood clotting after I hit the toe (should have come in then, should have gone somewhere at least), only cuts the nail down and gives me a local medication. It will take many months to remedy it, if indeed it can be fixed. Come in in four weeks. Fee: $43! All is relative. Instead of a black nail, I have no nail. Boring recital, I know, but my paying attention to it was a sign. Of health. Of optimism.

Not so the night. A bad one. It started earlier when Vic came home somewhat later than I expected and while I waited, I got an attack of nerves. Occasioned, of course, by that "friendly" warning I had received. It's three weeks now, my head tells me it was wrong, as did Vic, with chapter and verse, but still it haunts me, resurrecting old fears. Perfectly acceptable reason for his lateness, which wasn't even that, it's that he wasn't *early* as he had said he might be; a hurried dinner, then off to the theater. Cab driver, named Cohen, announced he was a "racist and a bigot," regaled us with his hate for Lindsay, and said he wished Lindsay's children had married "niggers," told us he thought little of Wagner too, and ended with "his wife, Susan, she was his brains, but then when she found out she had cancer, she became an alcoholic." Finally Vic managed to find a new subject—to wit, the workings of the publicity committee of the American Cancer Society whose meetings he is attending all this week. We go to their dinner Friday night—honored guest, Mrs. Ford. Does it bother him subliminally to be talking about it and working with them? I can't tell. I know it bothers me—not so much the subject but the necessity for acting impersonally about it and asking impersonal questions when now and then the whole subject appears to me as one large SCREAM.

To bed, and for some reason, the serpent insinuation insinuates again. I scold myself. It's not true, I know it, and still . . . I fall asleep, wake up to find Vic stirring and getting out of bed. What's troubling him? I don't ask him, although normally I would, because I suddenly wonder if he is being troubled by what is troubling me, and for the first time since spring and the last surgery, I break into a hot flash and sweat and suddenly I am furious at my "friend." (I have been worried about how to bridge the misunderstanding until now.) She did a wicked thing. Women, as we know, have killed, if only themselves, for that. But what makes me angriest—and that is why I feel honor-bound to put this into the record—is that I do not know what is going on inside me. I know it's a lie (know? Does one ever know anything? No, that much I *do* know), in my head and maybe even my heart, but that doesn't help the churning. And I do not want to hurt myself. I still have a feeling, unscientific though it may be, that I did this to myself (this? the cancer), and also have the feeling (I started to say "had" which proves my point) that my will to be healthy and live is helping me keep well, cancer-free. So I deeply resent and fear anything that upsets my subconscious where I have no conscious control. Nothing Vic can do about it. I even talked to him about it a little on Sunday, but how can he disprove something that isn't (he says)? "That's your problem," he said reasonably, and I know it.

So I lie awake while Vic reads in the other room and try to make a story out of it. Turn it into a chapter of something in my mind (note—as I write, my left eye has developed a tic), and finally manage to get so much out of it, at three a.m. (by morning, alas, it has all pretty much vanished), that I am almost happy again. Vic returns but I pretend I am asleep. Still can't talk to him. In the morning I mention he has had a bad night. He agrees. He had a nightmare—of Kim being raped and his pursuing the rapist. Our racist cab driver maybe; our walk up a frighteningly pornographic Broadway after the play. I am reading Jung on dreams and I remember his saying a dream can mean just what it says, so I hesitate to make analyses. Oddly enough I have just had a dream about Kim, too (rare for me to dream about her, I'm not sure I ever did before). In this one I am looking for passports for her and Polly because Vic is going to take them on a trip; I don't find the passports but I do find stocks made out to Kim, and our wills, new ones apparently, at which I decide not to look. Before Vic woke up I had been trying to figure out the Kim dream. Anger because I want to go away and he is taking them instead? Anger because they are able to go away while I am trapped? I don't know. In the light of morning I am angry at myself for having been angry at Vic—what did he do? nothing—and anguished because he is so harassed. Later, swimming, I think of his dream. Is Kim a symbol of someone else? Is that what goes on with the Cancer Society meetings? I swim some more and I tell myself—and believe it—that even if he does make a call or have a drink (which he may—I would were I he, if only to prove to myself that I'm not a bastard, and also because he has so few real friends, every one is precious), it has nothing to do with me at all. As he once said, I have 99 percent, why must I clutch at the 1 percent?

Easier said than accepted. Back home I look at myself in the mirror. Is he glad to have me around? Am I a strain? A burden? Is it in his mind as much as it is in mine?

I try to reverse positions. Would it be a strain, waiting for the shoe to fall? Yes. A burden? No. I think he would be more precious.

As I have felt myself to be all along—until that goddamned remark.

The only thing that makes it bearable is my knowledge that this, too, will pass. Be suppressed. Fade away.

Strange, I could take so much before, and even an insinuation is too much for me now.

November 7. That tempest passed. Dinner party Wednesday, calm and serene. Lunch and a concert yesterday. This morning at six I awoke in a sweat, remembered that I have been hot for days and that Vic yesterday, kissing me when he came home, said I was steaming. Is it possible the upheaval was soma, rather than psyche? My feet are somewhat swollen so I have trouble even with the larger shoes I bought (it's still warm out), and I've had a sort of pre-menstrual headache for days. There's something hormonal—a pile-up of hormones, or lack of some, I have no idea—and having named it, I felt—and feel—better yet. All I have to do this week-end is watch not to get upset by my body and confuse it with my mind, or heart.

Why should it be comforting to have the body upset rather than the mind? Why? The reason is obvious. But also funny. The body feels apart, someone else, over whom I have no control, therefore no blame, but my mind is me, even to the extent of be-ing ungrammatical.

The Philharmonic concert was very exciting. First concert we have been to in years. Essentially we have tin ears, I think. But this time something seemed to have happened to me. My mind wan-dered very little, and for the first time, I seemed to *feel* what Beethoven and Barber were feeling. Beethoven saying what I sense inchoately with a grandeur I only grasp at; Barber, to me at least, alternating a love of the beauty and delicacy of the world with shrieking rage at its inequities. I had a sense of release when the orchestra reached its crescendos—and a sense of order and gran-deur in the Beethoven that was very comforting. Words. What I am trying to express is the feeling I had listening to the music that I lead a very passionate inner life these days that I cannot put into words, much less share with anyone, and that that is what the sym-phony and the concerto were all about. I left, not tired, but exalted —and we walked to the bus on Ninth Avenue, bought pastrami sandwiches, and brought them home and ate them with mugs of beer.

Now-ness. Is-ness.
Goethe: "Do not, I beg of you, look for anything beyond phenomena. They are themselves their own lesson."

Joshu, asked what was the Tao, or truth, of Zen, said: "Your everyday life, that is the Tao."

> The morning glory blooms but an hour
> And yet it differs not at heart
> From the giant pine that lives
> For a thousand years.

"Who is God? I can think of no better answer than, He who is." St. Bernard.

Beethoven and beer.

Jung, at eighty-three, ten days before he died, on religious belief: "And how do we know that such ideas are not true? Many people would agree with me if I stated flatly that such ideas are probably illusions. What they fail to realize is that the denial is as impossible to 'prove' as the assertion of religious belief. We are entirely free to choose which point of view we take; it will in any case be an arbitrary decision.

"There is, however, a strong empirical reason why we should cultivate thoughts that can never be proved. It is that they are known to be useful. Man positively needs general ideas and convictions that will give a meaning to his life and enable him to find a place for himself in the universe. He can stand the most incredible hardships when he is convinced that they make sense; he is crushed when, on top of all his misfortunes, he has to admit that he is taking part in a 'tale told by an idiot.' "

Anything I try to write seems trivial—or rather, the writing itself seems trivial—compared to the depths from which the themes come.

Maybe I was able to hear the music because I was able to grasp the notes, one by one, in the here and now, each one emerging in time, in the moment, past notes vanished, future notes non-existent, alive only to what could be heard in the present. Carpe momentum. It tears me apart with joy.

A journal is a leap of faith. You write without knowing what the next day's entry will be—or when the last.

November 8. Up betimes, and the American Cancer Society annual dinner at the Waldorf. Full of Southern Wasps, retired doctors, and earnest ladies in long dresses. En route to the bar was met by a lovely-looking woman about my age, I suppose, who admired my necklace and introduced herself as something Perkins. From Missouri. I, in turn, admired her necklace, said it looked Nepalese, was told it came from Africa. A Koran holder, but empty. After making conversation for a while, she said she was a new director of the Society, and "one of the walking wounded." I looked at her. No sign of anything. Mastectomy? Maybe. No way of telling. What was I to say? I didn't, asked instead what else she did. "Save wolves," she answered. As, indeed, she does. There is a wolf sanctuary in St. Louis, she explained. First I asked why, then took back the question. Why not? Instead I suggested she put something from Job in her empty Koran holder. Something about God making Behemoth, the foundation of the earth, probably wolves. (Mystery was later solved when someone said her husband ran the zoo and was a television producer of wildlife films. Perkins himself.) Fleeting thought—organize a unit to save hyenas. We are all children of the Lord. Every last cell of us.

Then to the dinner. Hundreds of people, Mrs. Ford, Secret Service, much good cheer about cancer. Was boggled when an Episcopalian priest in his invocation asked God to help all "the good people here" in their good fight against the "scourge." Wouldn't it be simpler if God forgot the intermediaries and just didn't have it to begin with? Was boggled again when he gave a final parting blessing and confided to all of us that his father had been "cursed with cancer," sounded that way anyhow, and that in his name and God's, he was wishing that "the light of His countenance shine upon you," etc.

In between we heard the leading French oncologist, head of the international equivalent of ACS, speak of the fight against "cahnsay," a much pleasanter pronunciation; Johnny Bench, baseball star, speak of his "brush" with cancer (not so—a benign tumor, it was) and a four-year-old friend of his who had died of leukemia the day after telling his mother "baby Jesus wanted to see him"; Flip Wilson, and Mrs. Ford, who said she had just had her annual checkup, felt "marvelous," was found to be "cancer-free," and was "sure" she was cured. She said her only problem after surgery had been to cheer up her husband and children, who were terribly depressed about it all. The only place she retreated from her prepared script, which someone at our table had, was to insert—"at present"—in one of her disavowals. Fascinating speech —between the lines—because she did not speak of fear, mutilation ("I asked myself which I would rather lose, a right arm, or a right breast, and of course, I picked a breast"), the need for family understanding, but all of it in a kind of reverse logic. She also made clear what makes it bearable for her—her conviction that she has saved innumerable lives by her own candor, i.e., there is a "reason for it all."

Meanwhile, at our table sat a young man and his young wife, newly married, because he is now "symptom-free" of leukemia. He smoked.

It was like something out of *Alice in Wonderland;* the dinner, the flowers, the band playing dance tunes, State songs; the football cheer atmosphere, "Let's have it for cancer, boys!"

I felt quite removed from it all. And had ABSOLUTELY no desire or compulsion to confide that I was a club member, too.

None of it seemed to me to have anything to do with the reality of how anyone copes.

I guess I'm unfair. They do give grants. They raise money. And the ladies in long dresses probably drive patients, man booths, give out coffee in waiting rooms. At least I hope they do. Which is more than I do.

Series 9

November 11. I shouldn't write this today, I should be at something else, but today reminds me of the story about Voltaire that my mother loved so much (I told it to her, but it was one of the last stories she told me, and it fit). It's about Voltaire making a suicide pact with a friend, but when the friend turned up at Ferney at the agreed-upon time, he found Voltaire polishing off a croissant in the garden and looking overjoyed. The friend inquired what was up. "Oh," said Voltaire, "it's true, I was going to kill myself, but that was before my bowels moved." Which brings me to yesterday . . .

The weekend was amiable, but fraught. After the dinner, we went up to the country and while Vic slept in the afternoon, I waited for my sisters-in-law Mollie and Edith to turn up with the kids. They didn't until five, and then it turned out that Edith's car had been wrecked with the children in the back seat, and, while everyone was all right, Edith was shaken, and so were we, hearing. (The impact grew—even now, I see those dearly beloved faces, and I can't absorb it. It happened to someone else, not to Kim and Polly. I know, they're okay, but . . .) Then, a half hour later, came the call from Rhinebeck—the project plummeted. Again. How Vic keeps his resilience . . . ? Well, this time, fortunately in a way, he showed it. We played bridge, he slept . . . the weekend passed.

At seven, in the rain, I set out for Mark's. Too early, but I was afraid of missing the bus, and anyway, I hadn't been able to sleep (Vic did, finally, having taken a Valium, his first I think in maybe a year—each time, after my surgery, he did . . .). I told Mark about Rhinebeck, pertinent to this, because I realize that some of the uncertainty in these pages may stem from our actual living status—from week to week, we just do not know, or at least Vic doesn't, and I ache for him . . . I also told him of my pain about my friend, and his advice was instant, and obvious, and right . . . if we can do it. So, feeling relieved, I made the rain-swept journey down, went swimming briefly, marketed, ate lunch, and suddenly felt so tired I did something I have not done since I got out of the hospital, took the phone off the hook.

That was at two. At five I woke up, ate something, read a little, went back to sleep. And slept, with only a few interruptions, around the clock until eight o'clock this morning! (One interruption, Vic from Skokie—the Rhinebeck board still likes the idea, maybe they'll do something about it, but the Skokie thing is in abeyance . . . another, at eleven, was Kathy—her brain scan showed a physiological, but not a pathological, something, I really couldn't follow, except resolutely to put it out of my mind, she sounded relieved, so am I, it has to be a case of everyone knowing too much, I know, denial, denial . . .)

Anyhow—

This morning I am ebullient, joyous, well, optimistic . . . even resisted taking the Alkeran for a moment—not me, bud, wrong person . . .

For almost a day I stopped the world and got off (while I was sleeping the UN voted its infamous Zionist resolution, Jane tells me, and God knows what else happened, but *I* wasn't around).

And you know what?

I just realized that for the first time since I can't remember, my bowels haven't moved this morning.

A koan.

Very Zen.

Love to the world.

If only I could write the books I tell myself at three o'clock in the morning! The latest has a great dedication—"To Julie's great-great-grandchildren—Kim, Polly and Benjamin (at least)."

November 12. "A name is not a diagnosis. It does not determine treatment. Its original purpose, perhaps, was to distinguish between wise and foolish expectations, but its net effect has come to be that of destroying hope."

" 'Worse than despair, worse than the bitterness of death, is hope' (Shelley), or 'Hope is the worst of evils, for it prolongs the torment of man' (Nietzsche)—I have had some patients who agreed with these poets. Partly that is why they were patients."

"Confirmation for the sustaining function of hope in life has recently come from a most unexpected quarter—the psychobiological laboratory . . . When placed in certain situations which seemed to permit no chance for escape, even vigorous animals gave up their efforts and rapidly succumbed to death. . . . After elimination of the hopelessness feature . . . a rat that would certainly have died in another minute or two, becomes normally active and aggressive, swimming vigorously for fifty to sixty hours . . ."

The above, excerpts from a speech delivered by Dr. Karl Menninger fifteen years ago, reprinted in the pamphlet accompanying the fiftieth anniversary Menninger Clinic convocation at the Waldorf yesterday. To which I went—with Vic—expecting to find wisdom. All I found was the reprint—for the rest not one of the speakers said anything worth reflecting upon or remembering. The most interesting revelation came in the hallway when Ed Rosenthal interrupted my marveling at how wonderful it must have been for the family to work together so fruitfully to tell me that Drs. Karl and Will feuded so violently that Dr. Will couldn't spend time in Topeka and went proselytizing instead. That's a marvel in its way, too—more of "heed the philosophy, not the philosopher?" It truly puzzles me.

. . . The weather has cooled and I feel almost slim. Zippers zip, rings slip on. You're welcome.

November 13. Phenomenon:
I made arrangements to go to the country and when I mentioned the time, Margit said, "How about your test?"

"What test?" I asked.

"Your test," she repeated.

"My God," I said. "I forgot about the lab. I guess I'd better go first."

First time since I began chemotherapy.

I'm delighted.

November 15. From *The Ascent of Man:*
"There is no absolute knowledge. And those who claim it, whether they are scientists or dogmatists, open the door to tragedy. All information is imperfect. We have to treat it with humility. That is the human condition; and that is what quantum physics says. I mean that literally."

On Heisenberg's Principle of Uncertainty: "We should call it the Principle of Tolerance. And I propose that name in two senses. First, in the engineering sense. Science has progressed step by step, the most successful enterprise in the ascent of man, because it has understood that the exchange of information between man and nature, and man and man, can only take place with a certain tolerance. But second, I also use the word passionately about the real world. All knowledge, all information between human beings can only be exchanged within a play of tolerance. And that is true whether the exchange is in science, or in literature, or in religion, or in politics, or even in any form of thought that aspires to dogma." Blessed uncertainty.

On Einstein: "Einstein was a man who could ask immensely simple questions. And what his life showed, and his work, is that when the answers are simple too, then you hear God thinking."

The man to whom we "owe the fact that the atom—the world within a world—is as real to us now as our own world," Ludwig Boltzmann, "at the age of sixty-two, feeling isolated and defeated, at the very moment atomic doctrine was going to win, . . . thought all was lost, and . . . committed suicide."

The last paragraph: "We are all afraid, for our confidence, for the future, for the world. That is the nature of the human imagination. Yet every man, every civilization, has gone forward because of its engagement with what it has set itself to do."

The jacket says, "Jacob Bronowski died suddenly August 22, 1974."

What strikes me is what a pity he didn't have time—foreknowledge. What a man like that could have thought, knowing in his very cells that his time was limited! Of course, he *knew*—but not in the same way. I am sure he would have found a Machu Picchu inside him, the blue glow of the neutron shining over his desk. On second thought, looking at his face on the dust jacket, I guess he did know already. As he intimated, the scientist has an intuition about what he is looking for.

Anyway—at this moment—Saturday, November 15—to have missed this particular journey, bumps, heat, arid stretches, fearful descents notwithstanding, would seem a deprivation.

Woke up with a dream this morning. Disturbing in some ways—I was back in college, lost, feeling friendless, involved with an essentially uncaring young man (!)—but what was interesting about it was that it was the same dream I had a while back after surgery, I forget which one—and then the dream ended with my saying, "But I've been through all that. I don't have to go through it. I have cancer." No more.

Of a piece with my forgetting to have my blood checked yesterday?

Also noteworthy: No sense that the evil eye was going to

strike me for noting same. Kiddo, in the face of reality, you're just
a child's bogeyman! Another card, said Alice.

Called by the Knopf publicity woman. Read the galleys,
thinks the book is best thing I've ever done, qualitatively different.
"I just loved it, we're going to try to do good things with it."
"Thank you," I said. "I hope so."

Five minutes later, Gottlieb's assistant, Martha Kaplan, called.
"Good news. Literary Guild is taking it. As an alternate. You
ought to be so happy!" "That's nice," I said. "It would be better if
it were the main selection though." What is happening to me?

Such ups and downs. Subliminally the depression occasioned
by the "friendly" warning persists. Vic senses it—keeps me moving, so we went walking Sunday in Peekskill, then drove up to
Cold Spring for lunch, went into the city to have dinner with Jan.
Monday we went to Rhinebeck—normally I wouldn't go to a
Chamber of Commerce meeting, but it seemed a good idea. Tuesday, theater. Should be enough, but still today I woke up from a
nightmare about his upcoming trip to Los Angeles, and fought the
demons all morning. He invited me to lunch but I called to tell
him he didn't have to, I was fine. He called thereafter several
times to tell me about Rhinebeck—first off, now, dammit, on
again—finally asked me if I was all right. This time I told him
what was bothering me—not that it is true, I hurried to say, or
that I want to know if it is, or even that it is important, etc., etc.—
the feeling just is. His reaction: unfeigned bewilderment and reassurance. Not anger. So it went—and left me limp.

Later I went to swim—to see if I could exorcise the demon
by moving—and some poignant love song over the Muzak made
me wonder. I never really reacted to menopause, and certainly not
to the hysterectomy, in the sense that I felt middle-aged, or old, or
graying (which I am), or less attractive than I ever feel (that is,
my insecurities weren't greater, if anything, they were less—sometimes). Maybe I am mourning—the word stops me cold now—I
didn't mean it to come out—it just did—that is what I am doing.
Mourning. I look up, and I have a picture of a Shade in my mind,

something Greek or Roman, a funeral bas-relief, me. I am a Shade
dwelling in their midst, on loan, temporary, past. Not cancer so
much as sixty, I think, but maybe not. Maybe because of the cancer
I can't have the mental picture of the lusty healthy onward-and-
upward person I carried with me. And that's funny too, rereading
that last line. "Lusty?" "Onward and upward?" That's the self-
image I had? Of course not. But I think what I did have is a kind
of expanding universe feeling, that's true, of myself getting older
in a very positive sense, bigger (well, that I'm doing!), easier,
more open, healthy, certainly healthy. Well, that I don't have.
Note: These are today's ruminations, at five p.m., on a dreary day
—tonight's, tomorrow's, I know, *may* be, *will* be different.) I feel
as if I am someone diminished to live with, and it pains me. I don't
see us going off joyously into the sunset, just venturing timidly
step by step, and I hate it, and I hate anything that reminds me
that nothing is perfect or entire or whole . . . The words we use
to mask jealousy . . . but I may be unfair, as I have said, unfair
to myself, I mean, because it may not be jealousy disguised at all,
but a reason for mourning. I feel INTERIM.

Does saying it help? I hope so. I'm not sure. Because it happens to be true. I think. How do I know really? I don't.

Sunday night Jan startled me. I asked her if she wanted to do
Christmas, because we take the kids the next day, and she said yes.
Then added, "This year I'll be able to cook. Last year I was so
upset." I looked at her. Of course. Quiet, churning Jan. So that
Christmas Day when I thought I was being so noble and secretive
they were all suffering. I am swept by a pain so overwhelming I
can't bear it. I don't want them to be hurt by me, I don't want
them to have to go through it! I make a wish driving back—let
me be well through Christmas, through the book, through the
baby—oh, nuts, let me be well.

What have I done with this day? I should be ashamed of myself. I squandered it, conjuring up ghosts, wrestling with shadows.

Shame on me. Somewhere in opera there is a Dance of the Happy Shades. If you're going to be a shade, at least be a happy one.

November 20. I have decided that this journal, like most things, is two-pronged. As a device for self-knowledge, letting off steam (or vapors), and an illusion of usefulness (not an illusion —it is), it's fine. But it is also an accessory in self-consciousness, and morbid, tending to freeze what might melt with the instant. At any rate, I have avoided it for the last few days.

Vic came in as I was finishing the last entry and caught me by surprise, so much so that I read it to him by way of explaining my jumpiness of the last few days. It was a calculated risk—I knew it would trouble him, but again, lack of sharing is troublesome, too. But it's unfair. He felt pinned against a wall, helpless, frustrated. I tried to tell him of the double "journey" I take, and of its joys as well as its sorrows, but he couldn't absorb it. All he could say was, "I don't know what to do, I feel helpless, what can I say?" I told him I didn't want him to "say," just to share, but unless he can "do," he is at a loss. (The precipitating incident got lost in the discussion—and has remained lost to this day—which, I suppose, is what, deep down, I wanted to happen.)

The result was that he stepped up his phone-calling (four or five times the next morning, with anecdote, progress report on Rhinebeck, change of plan, etc.), got theater tickets for Wednesday (he had already gotten them for Tuesday), kept "doing" as much as he could by way of reassurance until I wanted to say "enough." But that is his way of coping, and I suppose I needed it, because I am all right now.

I have also been keeping busy—outside of the house (my old dilemma—I have to be alone to work, or even think about work, and if I am alone too long, I get ingrown. No solution except what I do—when it gets too much, I start moving. Not unique, either, all people who work alone have the problem). And as always, I am amazed that when I reach out, there *are* things to do, and people to talk to. I just have to be reminded that the choice is mine.

Finally made a breakthrough with Mary, the girl who does my blood at Jetti Katz. Alas. She asked me if I was going to have my "treatment" soon, and when I told her Monday, as usual, she said, "Good. I was worried about you. Your white count was very low last time." Maybe she said "low," not "very low," I don't really remember. My "treatment," of course, doesn't help the count, but I didn't tell her so. I just felt faint and frail as I walked down the street. Naturally. Obviously that's why I'm being watched, and I assume that Mark can cut down the pills even more. It makes me think about the chemotherapy though. My nails are splitting. My hair line is dry. Is it getting to me? If so, does it get stopped? *When* does it get stopped? *Does* it get stopped, by design, not by life? I realize it feels like a shield to me. I don't enjoy the pinpricks or the sense I have of everyone weighing balances around me, but it does represent security to me. As usual, anticipating, I wonder how I would feel if it were stopped—relieved, victorious (one more step of the battle won), or naked unto mine enemies? Okay. Not my decision. I'm not brooding over it, that's for sure, it's just one more observation.

Saw my wax lady again. She looks like a frail, beautiful, gentle Gabor sister. I don't know what happens between us, but something does. This time she talked about Auschwitz—she was very young, and must have been very beautiful, and I shudder to think how she, out of two sisters, two brothers and two parents, survived—and the deep depression that has to shadow one's life after having been through such an experience. Again I try— nothing redeeming? From talking about Israel and the anti-Zionist resolution and the horror it must be for parents who themselves suffered so much to have their children on the front lines we get something—her utter consuming devotion to her own two. (Not her husband, strangely.) When I leave, she touches me. "I am so very happy to have you here," she says, and I have to hold on to myself to keep from embracing her. I haven't said anything to her but we are communicating nevertheless on a very deep level.

Telephone busy all morning, with plans for Thanksgiving and Christmas. Jan, Kathy, Edith, Mollie, etc., and I get a pang. Please, please, don't let me spoil it for anyone!

(Life swirls. Vic brings me tea! Then he leaves me to this. I turn in my chair, catch a glimpse of that last smiling picture of my mother, and I long to see her. I miss her dreadfully suddenly, and I am very happy about that! And am reminded of Hokusai, who said he refused to paint shadows. But it's all light and dark.)

And now to my friend Hadrian. Mark told me to look at the book. I finally found it on the discard pile in the Bedford Hills Library (no bookstore had it in stock). I remembered the story well enough. I saw Antinoüs in Egypt, I think, and certainly at the Villa. But the dying—not at all. With joy I come upon the first chapter—"It is difficult to remain an emperor in the presence of a physician, and difficult even to keep one's essential quality as a man." Exactly. The difference between Dr. Bulkin, whom I didn't know, and Mark, who knows me now.

Beautiful quotations—"I am not yet weak enough to yield to fearful imaginings, which are almost as absurd as illusions of hope, and are certainly harder to bear. If I must deceive myself, I should prefer to stay on the side of confidence, for I shall lose no more there and shall suffer less . . . To say that my days are numbered signifies nothing; they always were, and are so for us all. But uncertainty as to the place, the time, and the manner, which keeps us from distinguishing the goal toward which we continually advance, diminishes for me with the progress of my fatal malady. A man may die at any hour, but a sick man knows that he will no longer be alive in ten years' time." Ten years. Interesting figure. Mine, deep down. It's all so convincing that I keep forgetting it isn't Hadrian but Marguerite Yourcenar speaking.

Bits—Trajan sitting on the shore of the Persian Gulf, weeping, for the first time "confronting his own life face to face."

Hadrian, like Alexander, making "a sacrifice to Fear before entering into Rome." I had the references in *Mrs. Beneker,* I think, but I don't think I understood the Fear he mentioned then. Somewhere in the book, too, he (or Yourcenar) mentions that his every other thought is of his own death, and he adds, "Meditation upon death does not teach one how to die . . ."

Hadrian was, of course, dying. I, I must remind myself, am not. As Mark said weeks ago, I tend to get confused about my present. And as I noted at the start of this notation, this journal, if I am not careful, adds to the confusion. I must remember, it is *not* a journal about living with cancer, it is a journal about living with *chemotherapy* which is a constant reminder of cancer. The canker, once removed.

November 21. Relaxed with Cyril Connolly's *The Evening Colonnade.* First essay: Aldous Huxley. First paragraph: "O miserable and fatuous humanity which still squanders on armaments and space trips the fortunes which might help to find a cure of the most ruthless, painful and humiliating of ailments, that destroys the finest minds and bodies in their prime and denies old age the privilege of natural death!"

Ah, so.

In fairness, another quotation, from Laura Huxley: "There are two diametrically opposite views about dying. One is that the best way is to go without knowing it, to slip away—hopefully when sleeping. The other view is that one should die as aware and clear-minded as possible: that death is one of the great adventures of life. Aldous believed in the latter."

Well, he did finish an essay three days before he died—"in great pain," says Connolly—and he used psychedelics to numb his body.

I turn therefore to Hemingway and on the first page come

upon—"Any man who allowed himself to suffer from women had a disease as incurable as cancer."

Nuts.

Why is everyone so obsessed?

(Don't tell me—I know—but there is a black humor in it all the same, wherever I run to, someone stands ready to turn me around and rub my nose in it . . .)

November 22. The mind is a place in itself.

Saw Mark and mentioned the white count. He showed me the figures. Up, not down, the last two weeks. Other bloods fine. All of them higher than when I started. (It was post-surgery, of course, but even so . . .) Immediately I get mystical. Something in me. Will to live. Mirror-image of my perhaps not having wished to live. (Not so far-fetched really. I remember a weekend when Vic had left me when I decided not to drive. I was making too many left turns without looking in my mirror.) Well, as Hadrian would say, a constructive fantasy. I had a sudden flash of my sister—and my mother—and their prayers answered. Oh, dear.

But I feel different. Reprieved somehow. And there is another reason for it. Mark said I would have a chest X-ray in January. Period. Let sleeping dogs lie. I have been so apprehensive about going through another series of tests, repeating last December. (I know. Evil eye. A very small effigy still, no bigger than a child's puppet.)

. . . My agent Anne just called. Where is that article I had promised? It isn't. She asks me if I'm depressed. It turns out it's my voice—she isn't used to it being low. Then she tells me about a friend who has just had a mastectomy and has "two years to live." "They told her?" "Sure. I'd want to know." "Why?" I ask. "I would change my life," she says. "Stop working. Go to Europe. Do all the things I haven't done." I mention her husband, who has his work at Yale; her daughters, who are of school age. "I'd take them out of school." I guess she would. But I gently point out that it's easier said than done. "But you can live your life the way you want it," she says. Do I? I don't know. And I remember waking up in the middle of the night asking myself who I am, that childish question everyone seems to be asking. Not who I am, exactly. More—I am different than I used to be, but how I am, at times, a little unfamiliar to myself, but with all my mulling about and introspection, I never take time to figure it out. If indeed I can. I don't even know what I look like!

December 3. Just a few notes for the record. I have been absent from this journal for over a week now, by mutual agreement with myself. And I have been busy, also by agreement. It was time, and helpful.

Thanksgiving, of course, intervened, with children and grandchildren and family, and very lovely and peaceful, as all holidays have been since . . . I don't know whether everyone subliminally shares my gratitude or not, but the tensions have gone from holidays. We even had a birthday celebration for Vic, which he enjoyed, to the extent of being wistful about people not wishing him a happy birthday the day after (which was his real birthday), only I remembering. I smiled. In the past, we had to ignore his birthdays, or almost so, because they bothered him.

But it was good, and I was aware that another year has passed and I was making the stuffing and the cranberries and the walnut roll. Then Kathy and Hilary were negotiating over buying a house, and it finally came through, and I'm going to see it Friday. Also an event underlined by my presence. I can *mother* for another while —baby, house, etc.

Only sad note today (and Vic is in California, and that isn't sad at all, please note—I'm enjoying these days, I have filled them up and I like hacking around the apartment by myself at night—I have no bad feelings about it, except—to be honest—I did have one brief funny dream which was like a final mopping-up, and it amused and soothed me, it was so obvious)—anyway—the one sad note is that Jan last night confessed what she's known for a couple of weeks. She has to have a cyst removed from the end of her spine next Tuesday. In Mount Sinai, but as a day patient, and everyone assures her, but she was/is so scared of the unmentionable—"the doctor said I know what's been going on in your family, so don't worry, I'll do a biopsy, but he would have put me in right away if it was anything, wouldn't he?" she said. I'm upset she didn't think she could tell me earlier and sad, again, that she should be upset (that's why the Sunday dinners, and her mentioning her worry about me before!). I'm not worried that it's anything though. I just don't want them to have pain or worry! Especially through me.

December 4. Saw Ida yesterday, serene in her bed—"I'm eighty-five, and I have no pain," she managed to say. I looked at her. Usually I would have been sympathetic, now I'm envious.

—In bus en route I saw an old lady getting off and realized I won't be.

—In *Times* this a.m. estrogen seen as cause of uterine cancer —when I think of how I shopped around to get someone to prescribe it for me—that's what it amounted to, although I didn't say so out loud.

—What I am doing here is research for when I will need it —when I can't do it myself.

I have had a real sense of freedom not having the chemotherapy these past couple of weeks. It feels like a vacation, even though it really isn't a burden. I like seeing Mark. I like being around Madison Avenue to get my blood test. So . . .

.   .

Vic has finally noticed my weight. "You feel so *fluffy*," he said the other night, not displeased.

December 10. The date says the most there is to say. Another week away from the journal (and introspection). Something seems to have happened to me—AT THIS MOMENT—I am at peace. All week I have had the sense of doing only what I want to do, without pressure. I haven't been writing. So what. The world still moves, but more important, so do I. Vic's week away went well, and it was good to have him home again. I'm typing against the clock now, waiting to go to Knopf to assert myself about the publicity. Question—shall I say why I am so anxious for attention to be paid this time? I hope not.

Meanwhile, only notes. I have gone to the library some more, where I continue my secret research. Piling up material for the day when I may want to write but may not be able to go out and get what I want for myself, specifically, "how to do it." Huxley's letters, Laura Archera Huxley's account of his last days, Simone Weil, Bernanos, etc. The books are still in the library, and maybe I'll type out some quotes. But what I discovered is that the Huxley material, distilled through Sybille Bedford in her biography, comes out very hopeful and inspiring secondhand, but very sad and frightened in the original. He read from the Book of the Dead to his dying wife, and Laura, the second wife, tapes(!) his deathbed scenes and tries, oh, so obviously, to repeat his coup of the first death, and all it amounts to is babbling against the dark. I tried to track down an essay Huxley was said to have finished a few days before he died—"Shakespeare on Death," Connolly called it in his book—but all I could find in the files was "Shakespeare on Religion." Turns out that was the assignment, but Huxley concentrated so on Shakespeare's horror of death that it turned out to be Shakespeare on death. And he didn't *write* it, he put it on tape, phrase by phrase, with help, and with difficulty. No miracles. Not anywhere. Somehow I found the whole thing freeing, not frightening. As though there is a competition to see how well one does. (Incidentally I feel qualitatively different, stronger. Either time has passed since surgery—Bill Collins's magic "year"—or my psyche is in better shape. (Only a whiff of evil eye here, the shadow of the grin, like the Cheshire cat's.)

This search I am making pops out despite myself. Jackie had a big, big Sunday brunch, mostly people from Martha's Vineyard. Notably present was Albert Leventhal, who was literally given up for dead the weekend we were supposed to go to the Vineyard, and didn't because of my back (an excuse, anyway). So dire was his state, apparently, that the plugs were pulled—and he recovered on his own a week later! And is working every day now. And looks no jollier than he ever did. I remarked how well he seemed to Janice, whom I barely know, and then after a while of her talking, asked, "Is your life different now?" Meaning, of course, "What secrets have you found, etc., etc." Her response: "Oh, yes. We don't go out very much." I still didn't give up. "How does he feel?" I asked. "Serene?" "Oh, no," she said, "he gets very depressed." "And scared," I said, and she nodded. Time to stop, I guess. Or maybe not. It's sort of fun, an internal joke with myself, Candide peeking into Hades.

Also at the brunch, two women were talking about their difficulties about caring for their octogenarian mothers. I found myself thinking of myself as the troublesome mother, rather than the worried daughter, mostly because Jan's concern about telling me of her surgery still makes me uneasy. She's fine—surgery yesterday, she was home after four hours, I visited her today for a bit. Nothing. But said Lester, "They promised her they'd do a biopsy." (Fragment of a dream this morning—people upset because a doctor's wife named Greenberg miscarried. Jan and Kathy mixed together. In a way this mothering feeling I have is permission I give myself —I am well enough to hover—I will last long enough to budge— it's an opening-up, not a closing, although it may not look it. Just as my flying to Boston to see the house Hilary and Kathy are going to buy and making uncharacteristically positive remarks and suggestions was.)

Astonishments—in *Time* magazine, Paul Anka, thirty-four, "is thinking about what he hopes will be his next big hit: an album that will include songs about cancer and fear of dying." Maybe people are ready for a novel about same. If so, it will be about four years too early. I always am, although it is not so noticeable. All the books and plays about the McCarthy hearings now, and my chapters written five years ago went unnoticed.

—In *Times* magazine, magnificent interview with Ingmar Bergman in which he speaks of running "like a rabbit" until ten years ago when he stopped running and tried to find out about himself. He had a "minor operation," and "for five hours I was away, completely faded out, switched off. After that experience—the five hours that hadn't existed—I was no longer afraid of death. And everything that was outside this world no longer mattered. Since then I haven't thought about God."

Nor, adds he, has he thought of suicide, as he had before.

(Query: Is anesthesia so different from sleep? Does it affect the spirit as well as the body? I have had no experience of that. All I remember is the buried-alive terror of the first time when I was still a little conscious and my gratitude at not having been conscious when I woke up the second time.)

Also—"Koestler has a theory that the human brain is like a cancer," a mutation in a small monkey brain, "so mankind suffers from this cancer brain, this enormous, impractical thing we have to carry around over the little brain we need for our primitive simple functions." "Daffodils that come before the swallows dare"— the result of a cancer brain! $E = MC^2$? I'm sitting here trying to think of the loveliest lines I know and can't decide, but how marvelous! All the world's beauty some cells gone astray! As Bergman points out, "it is probably not true," but it's an enchanting idea.

I sold myself to the Knopf publicity man and did not mention *it,* only the "surgery" we had in common as the reason Sissman asked for the book.

December 11. Nine p.m. Vic out. So this really isn't taking refuge in the journal, it's just note-taking. Again I've been out all day. To Knopf, where my great coup of having them get a photographer for me has exploded. Terrible pictures. I either look like Lillian Hellman, which isn't the same as writing like her, or Alfred Knopf's wife, which is nice but still not me. They told me to go back to my family and have snapshots. Bob, back from his sales meeting in St. Martin's ("Horrible, the airport was like a blockaded seaport, with the Nazis strafing, and the Gestapo arranging for your cell"—he's still terrified of flying), says, "Someone said you were depressed, that you said this is probably the last book you're going to write. You can't do that to me, you owe me lots more books, after all I picked you up out of the gutter . . ." I smile. He knows what I meant, and that I was using it. Anyway I'm going to write him at least one more book. This one.

But it may not be very original. I went to Doubleday's to get some presents and found the front counter nearly jammed with titles such as *How to Live with Cancer, All About Cancer, How to Live with a Dying Husband,* etc. I'm not exaggerating at all. I looked at *How to Live . . .* but decided not to explore it. Too many jazzy case histories, every one terminal. Did get Kubler-Ross *On Death,* because it's a paperback, and cheap, and because it has a great bibliography for my secret library of necromania. Also bought a book about wine and a cookbook. Eat, drink, and be merry, right? Mostly Kubler-Ross talks about awareness of death as helping one to live in the present. Well, I'll tell you one thing I've noticed these last few days. I have been buying Christmas presents for everyone very serenely—quite literally as though there were no tomorrow—and it's the first time it's been fun. No sweat, no guilt (don't ask me why I used to be guilty about buying Christmas presents, I was, mostly because I thought I was inept, or every-thing was too expensive, or something). I am also finished, two weeks early. I also bought myself some clothes on sale. I've finally gone over the line—nothing of my size-8 past fits any more. Does it bother me? Not at all.

I do wonder whether I will ever have a figure again, but not too much. Because the question is fraught. *Why* will I get thin? For good reasons? Or for bad? Meanwhile, I buy larger pants, move buttons.

My breakthrough with Mary, the blood girl, continues. To-day she came in laughing and asked me where I had been. "I thought you were in last week, and then you weren't, it was some-one else, and I wondered . . ." I explained I was three on, three off. "Oh," she said. "Chemotherapy?" I nodded. "Aha," she said. "That's it." She looked at my head. "How is it you don't lose your hair? In the hospital . . ." "It's been nine months," I said, "I guess I won't." "But the patients I saw . . ." "I must be getting less," I said. It was better when she glowered.

Cheerful letter from my twenty-nine-year-old niece Joanna in answer to mine answering her request for word as to how I am:

"I'm glad you've been fighting off the cancer so well. It re-minds me of how whenever I get deathly ill, the doctors all tell me how healthy I am. Quite a few of my friends' mothers have cancer. I have a feeling that by the time my generation grows to be your age there will be a lot more of us."

À la mode, that's me.

Series 10

December 16. A metaphysical footnote, not so far removed from chemotherapy as one might think at first glance—the story of Ea.

I decided to do a little research on the Babylonian god Ea with the hope of possibly doing one of those "strange encounter" stories the Sunday *Times* travel section runs occasionally. But, for reasons which shall become apparent, it turns out to be too personal to be noted anywhere but here.

The episode goes back to the course I took in ancient Near Eastern religion the year Kathy had her strange illness. I have always had a good feeling about the statues to "unknown" gods some of the Near Eastern peoples included in their temples. The New Testament mentions one. And listening to the course lectures, I had moments of thinking that as an agnostic, I could accept a whole range of gods. I'm putting it pompously. I did it better in *Mrs. Beneker* when I fictionalized what actually did happen to me. She decides that some of the ancient gods might be left around and thinks up a guardian angel that looks a little like Harpo Marx. And when she hears her professor describe an incantation to a god named Ea, a Babylonian god, prayed to in sickness, she performs it. *"Shipta sha ea,"* accompanied by the pouring of water. She does it in a panic over her son critically injured in an auto accident; I did it in a panic the day Kathy was rushed to Montefiore and couldn't walk and had a spinal tap. Syncretism. When people have nothing to hang on to, nothing to believe in, they grasp at anything. Yoga. TM. Zen. Me, I picked a Sumerian demon adopted by Babylon. She got better, too.

Time passed. Eight years. On our first trip together after The Thing—to Iran, for me full of archaeology, a token by Vic—and we are still uneasy, or at least I am, wondering each time we check into a hotel, is he pleased to be with me?—and halfway through, we go to Pasargadae, near Persepolis, and somehow I wander away from the group and find myself alone near a strange god. Literally, a strange god. Alone and alien to Persia, a Babylonian fish god, the figure of a man with fish tail extremities, Ea himself. Put there thousands of years ago as a gesture. Not exactly an "unknown" god, but surely an alien one. I recognize him, and make a wish— which indeed comes true thereafter.

With this as my start, I got out Hooke's *Babylonian and Assyrian Religion* to see what I could make of it. I find that Ea's constellation is Pisces—I don't believe in astrology, but that's my sign. He is the god of healing, patron god of priests trained in knowledge of spells and incantations, exorcist of demons responsible for illness. The Babylonian *ashipu,* priest-doctor, always made sacrifices to Ea and called upon his intervention for the "sick man." The *ashipu* gave the sick a cake baked in the ashes sacrificed to Ea and buried an effigy in the desert, after which the afflicted person was regarded as risen from the dead, and a new man, healed.

Hooke also points out that each Babylonian god had a sacred number—Anu (their Zeus) had 60; Enlil (heaven) had 50; Ea had 40.

Forty is the number I found myself writing on my hand for no reason last fall. It's in the journal somewhere. As I remember, it was instrumental in solving what was a real crisis—for me. I just looked it up. It wasn't fall, it was June, but the number surely came out of nowhere.

Ea and Alkeran. Primitive, childish, and yet, Horatio—who knows?

December 23. This is probably my last—certainly my last typed—entry for the year, and it's curious how I've been avoiding this journal. I don't understand my reluctance except that I feel so *well*—in the sense of not feeling morbid—that I don't want to go near anything that reminds me that I am not, in fact, whole. If indeed, the journal does remind me.

"Well" isn't the word. "Normal" is more like it. And I got jogged today when the drugstore sent over the vial they had to get from the wholesaler for me (one of the two drugs Hilary is to inject Monday). I was jogged because it was over $21 for the dose, not only because I am suddenly aware of the value (literally and figuratively) of what I am being given, but because it must, ipso facto, be very special. Q.E.D.

I wonder what started the change. In part I think it was my library reading. It was so far overboard that I think I drowned and came up on the other side. As illustration, I had put in the calendar for next year a notice of a talk on "Death" at the White Institute by a Dr. Dahlberg. Ugh! I dumped it when I found it just now. It's like eating too much chocolate (and what a description of death literature that is—but it's accurate—that's what my wallowing was); you end up revolted. Good. That's a fine positive result, not to be confused with excursions into philosophy, which are life-enhancing, not destructive. (For now, at any rate.)

I found a note on a slip of paper just now—"Why the sudden calm? Because nothing has happened for a while?" The discomfort of being in equilibrium. Waiting for the shoe to fall. The fly to emerge. Evil eye, I guess, a few blinks to show it's still in the wings.

Other reasons. Flutterings about the book, all of them good, and flattering. I'm in the world again. Went to Toinette Rees's wedding and except for Anne McCormick and Gottlieb, I was the only Knopf or book person there. Also flattering, and very moving. I am pleased easily these days. Every gesture registers deeply.

And then, it's year's end, which is always a very profound time for me, and these years, doubly so. They mark anniversaries —two years from the first surgery, one year since the second—victories, really, or so they feel. I could have wept saying goodbye to Mark (a month this time, I hope, since Hilary does the last of this series for me), and could only mumble the commonplace, my gratitude and my love. Is he keeping me going? Sure, along with me, and Vic, yes, Vic, and Jan, and Kathy, and Jean, no question about it. Seltzer, I think that's his name, writing on surgery in *Harper's* this month tells of a man with a cancer eating a hole in his head who refused surgery month after month even though Seltzer told him he would get meningitis and die. One week he doesn't turn up, and then another. Seltzer goes to the luncheonette he owns to find out what has happened, and what has happened is pink skin over the hole in his head. Why? His sister-in-law brought a bottle of water from Lourdes and he washed the wound with it every day. "Holy water?" asks the surgeon. "Yep," says the man. I believe.

And so I've been counting my blessings, mostly people. (I kissed Mrs. Markham goodbye, too. Why? She didn't seem startled. She's part of my miracle, I feel that too. If only that she is the one doctor's wife I've encountered—and most of my best friends have been the same—who, far from resenting his patients, gives us the feeling she shares his feelings. At least so it seems to me. And must be herein writ as part of my year's end summing-up.) I made a little speech to Hattie, and one to Janet, who knew just what I meant because she made a little speech back to me. That's one of the year's treasures too. (It's odd how we know each other, we travelers on our road. At our friend Elmer's party I found a woman lawyer with outside characteristics, at least, paralleling ours— where we live, city and Florida; daughters, work, etc.—and inside of minutes I knew. Hers is a heart, as is Toinette's British mother, with whom, too, I had an instant rapport over and above community of interests, sharing of differences—her people came to London during the Spanish Inquisition, and she is going to be Mayoress of the Borough of Harrow of which she is now Councilperson, I love it—but underneath both of them was the current, carpe diem, enjoy, who knows?)

From L. E. Sissman's new book, a collection of essays:

Upon learning he has Hodgkin's: "It is like, I should imagine, being the first man to see for himself . . . the proof of the theory of the curvature of the earth." And, "I have been looking down at the curvature of the earth, at the trajectory of my life and death, from a new perspective: from the perspective of a tangential line lifting, straight as a contrail, away from the earth and myself and all the other things and people. It is, and has been, a lonely journey."

"Lonely?" Yes, and no. Or at least, lit, as I have said above, by the surprising little flashings of the lights of other travelers going the same road in the same darkness.

I think I shall end this entry with the note I found in the

back of last year's calendar: "May I end next year well—but as serene as I am now."—Jan. 1, 1975.

Puzzle for 1976? Why did I write "but" instead of "and"? Okay, why, as Gregory Zilboorg pointed out, did Freud misquote Shakespeare: "Thou owest Nature a death," he wrote, instead of "God." Herein a cigar is not a cigar.

What did I write for this year's notation: "I am well—and serene and I'm grateful."

Laude.

Back, Chest, and Tests

January 15, 1976. Having written the date I wanted to underline the year. So I did. I allow myself many freedoms these days.

However, I must say that pride goeth. My back is out. Not badly, but the other side, and I know *exactly* what started it. No tests, Mark dear. I was feeling so splendid—so strong—that Kathy complained in Sarasota. "How come you're the only one that doesn't get tired? The rest of us nap and collapse and you . . ." True. I made beds, washed dishes, cooked (they did too, everyone helped), used the rowing machine and bicycle machine in the house gym and swam in ice water (only Hilary, the kids, and I went in, not Vic and not anyone else in the whole apartment house, it was so cold and windy). Fine. Then we sublet the apartment and I took it apart—ten loads of laundry, lifting (Vic's back was out). Still okay. Then in front of the airport the car trunk wouldn't lift and when Kim pointed out what it was (while Vic went to get help), without thinking I jammed down the hood and snapped it open—and felt something in the area of my sacroiliac snap too. Long plane trip ensued. More bag lifting. And the coup de grace—the annual closet arranging in Mount Kisco. So FINALLY . . . It's not like the last time, and I took to my bed at once to keep it from being acute, but the three days bedded down until today (with time out for one dinner engagement I must confess, at which I felt not a twinge) have sobered me.

Because I had decided the last day in Sarasota, lying awake and writing in my head, which is the sign that something is beginning to cook, that again the mountain in my way of writing is this year, and I have to write it. Or should try. Not as a journal but as fiction (don't know of any book with this as a topic, but . . .) — and that, for this record, signified something. That I was beginning to be uninvolved in a sense—the experience was digested and outside me, if I may mix metaphors, and that I was ready to write it, encapsulate it, make it something that happened to someone else.

The first twinge of pain collapsed that house of cards (although the cards remain, I see that too—I shall pick them up and start over again, but the initial abandon is gone). And not because I think it's a cancer pain. Jan got upset when I told her I was lying down and said I should call "someone," and I told her right out: "It's not cancer, don't worry," "Okay," she said, relief obvious, and not denying what was in her mind. The pain is on the surface, it acts like a back, it subsides when I lie down, and it isn't much to begin with. Only for me, every twinge gives me a double-take, I realize. I get a gas pain in my chest and I think aha, angina, and I am pleased. (I am in an underlining mood today. Statements are so flat I am afraid the nuances get lost. Albert Leventhal, parenthetically, did die. In his sleep. How nice, I thought, especially since his wife was in London and not there to discover it.) I drop my hairbrush or spill a glass of water and think quietly, "Brain tumor." But this morning I saw Vic drop his hairbrush as he reached for it, and his pill box slipped, and I didn't think brain tumor, just "Oh, everyone drops things!"

A journal should be written almost daily. Otherwise the mood gets lost. It's hard for me now to get back to the sense of absolute well-ness and almost-forgetfulness I had. All I have is a few scraps of notes to remind me.

Re Kathy—Kathy, Hilary, Kim and Polly and Vic and I spent a week in a two-bedroom apartment without a murmur of dissent or discomfort. The whole holiday season was peaceful and lovely. Some of it unquestionably has to do with me. Kathy said casually that she said to Hilary when they were packing to come down, "This year I don't have to worry." Repeating Jan's remark that she was going to be able to cook this Christmas. Later she said she had been wondering whether my depression a couple of months back wasn't anticipatory—each of the two previous Christmas-New Year periods was marked by tests, anticipation, worry, surgery. Very likely. I don't know whether I verbalized it or not, but I do recall that being told that I only was going to need a chest X-ray this month made something lift in me. (Terrible the responsibility words and phrases represent, isn't it?) Also, when she asked me why I was being so energetic, I said, "Don't you see how glad I am to be able to do it?" And I was.

Re Hilary. The shots were very important to us both. He had brought a whole armament, including a gadget to hitch on to the intravenous needle, something with a little tube and smaller needle which eased the injection. He was very careful, very precise, very non-pain-causing. Odd footnote: As usual, a couple of hours after the injections, I suddenly got very tired. The tiredness lasted a half hour or so. I always thought it came from traveling from the Bronx and/or going to the pool right afterward, but this time, there was obviously no travel involved. Is it the injection or a psychological bracing and letdown of which I'm not aware?

I see a report in the *Times* saying some doctors in Texas have devised an almost foolproof test for cancer. My first reaction: "Good. Then they'll be able to tell if I have it." Second reaction: "Dope. You're on the other side of the line. You *have* it." But I don't believe it.

· ·

We go to hear Elie Wiesel speak. His topic: the Messiah. The auditorium is packed, people listening entranced. I wonder why. I know why I listen. His talk is a metaphor. For me. The Messiah is hope. We all wait, believing, not believing. It is hard to wait, harder not to wait. The waiting cannot be negative, but positive. The waiting time must be used advantageously. What sticks with me though is his quotation from Kafka which, I think, goes: The Messiah will not come on the last day, when hope is lost, but on the day after, when it is too late. That's as good a summary of what it is about as any—the world is divided into those who believe the Messiah will come in time, not at all, or too late.

I go through old papers and magazines, trying to catch up. Two I clip—"Cancer as a Metaphor for Death," in the January 4 Sunday *Times.* I read it on two levels—anguish—"No one wants to die of cancer or witness the pain and agony of others who are ravaged by it"—and literary interest—"We are concerned with our own mortality, and cancer is the contemporary symbol of our finiteness." The latter is why I want to write a novel, not the last year as cancer-haunted, but as a metaphor for life itself. "The ultimate cause of death is life." Everyone's cause of death.

The second is from *Newsweek*—a daughter's story of her father's death from cancer. No fun. Even "the trauma of an old World War I rifle that would not fire—a plastic bag . . . clawed away at the last minute . . . spilled pills." I think what amazes me most is that he was seventy-five. Seventy-five! Even then, trying with a rifle . . . Anyway, it does end on a note of grace. "A great elation."

My brushes with survivors continue. This time the woman behind the counter at the Éclair. Seen her on and off for six years. This time for no reason except that it is cold outside she tells me how she lived in Siberia in a Russian prison camp during World

War II. She tells me all the details—her father unable to bear it more than six months, her grandparents dying, the DP camps, her husband-to-be weighing eighty pounds and left for dead in Malthausen, her determination to live—"imagine, a girl of fourteen felling trees at forty below zero, even the Mongols felt sorry for me"—on and on. What has the most ring of truth is her confession: "You know, you never feel sorry for anyone else when you're going through it. My father died, my grandmother, my mother in prison, nothing made an impression. All I was interested in was myself. It took me years . . ." A beautiful excerpt on the concentration camps in this month's *Harper's* says, "The survivor stays alive in body and spirit, enduring dread and hopelessness without the loss of will to carry on in human ways."

Alas, he jests at scars. I can be philosophical so long as it's out there—with nary a twinge to remind me. Do I accept? Do I deny? Do I make much too much ado? Is it possible totally to ignore? I doubt the latter, but of the other three, I just don't know.

February 3. Back to the journal. Only in discomfort apparently. The past few weeks have vanished. A while back, a week or a little more of flu, and bed, bed, bed. Not so much a depression as a flatness. I couldn't wait to get going on life again this week.

But Monday began with a blizzard, and Mark home in bed, and today, Tuesday, I am to see Doctor Bulkin and have X-rays, chest and back. And how do I feel? With the whole episode "past," "encapsulated," "ready to be written about"? In a panic.

Vic saw my face when Mark said I was to have the X-rays, and became upset himself. "Why?" he asked. Why, indeed? I tried to explain. Anything that upsets the routine—even someone else giving me the shots—is upsetting. It's as though I have the thing pegged—and as long as everything is in its slot, I can operate around it. But if the pegs get moved . . .

On the other hand, Mark once said it is natural to get upset. Obviously the reason for X-rays is to find out if there is something.

My chest feels okay, my back pains seem to act like back pains, darting, inconsistent, but . . . even so.

So I worry, and hope I won't have to worry tomorrow. I began to go through the ritual—it can't be much if it is anything, after all I have no symptoms, but I can't do that to myself any more. I didn't have symptoms each time before either, and I do have one symptom—pain. What is, is. Only why do I always have this sense of disappointment about myself and my inability to breeze through this? More than disappointment—anger that I haven't used every minute, every golden minute *without pain,* to its utmost. I was right about trying to write it before it goes. It seems to me the highs are gone (did they exist, or was I fooling myself? I think they did), and now it's a matter of slogging through. It may, of course, just be winter, and the flu, and the back (I've had more trouble with that than anything, haven't I?)—the plateau.

I think I'm scared of the book, too. I can't imagine it being anything, although I guess I fantasize that, too, and if it is, I don't know if I'm up to it. But the world is full of books. Even a two-column review in Sunday's book review of a Knopf novel by a woman unknown to me adds up to nothing. So it comes out. A small firecracker in a tiny field. Pop. So what. What *is* important? To be content with each day. To *use* time. Which I haven't been doing. Tomorrow—when I don't have fever. Tomorrow—when the back is easier. Tomorrow—and today is tomorrow.

(Re the flu—I have rarely been sick before these last two years, and I'm not sure that the—I'm stuck for words again—the what? the cancer? I suppose so—should be classified as sickness. No? Why not? Okay, okay. Chronic, acute, I know the difference. Anyway I treated myself as an invalid and so did everyone else—Vic, Mark, etc.—with the sense that I am more vulnerable now. And felt it something of a victory that I did get over it quickly. Good white blood cells. Something like that. But it was a strange feeling nevertheless, to feel less than tough. I also have the feeling

that there is something wrong in accepting the vulnerability. It's
giving in.)

I WANT TO BREAK OUT. Swim. Exercise. Do. I haven't
even used the library for six weeks.

Well, let's get through today.

Tomorrow.

February 4.

A Mini-Drama.

Mark's office arranges for me to have the X-rays before my
shots today. Fine. That's how tests should be scheduled, I think—
at once, so you don't have time to brood about them. The girl in
the office, Barbara, couldn't be nicer. She is allowing an hour or
so for the tests, but of course they'll be over sooner.

Hah!

Nothing, as may have been noted before, is simple.

It begins with my father calling—at one-thirty in the afternoon—to find out how I am. Unprecedented. Why? Does his heart
know something I don't? I am touched—and apprehensive. (Typical—always superstition enters in when there is any question at all.)

I am taken at once by X-ray, and something immediately appears to be wrong with the chest X-ray. Naturally. The one X-ray I
could take in my stride. An hour and a half later, after Mr. Cohen,
the technician, has been in and out with boards for me to lie on,
and deep breaths for me to take (which, it turns out, I can't—that
pain in my right chest bone that made me sit up every time I had
to cough but somehow ignored apparently isn't in my head, or gas,
but SOMETHING), I am told I can go. "Did they find something?" He nods. "A tumor?" What else should I ask? "Don't look
for *tsouris,*" he says. He has long since recalled that he has done
me before, several times. Then he relents. "The pictures with
boards are to look for fluid usually," he says. "I had flu," I say.
"So," he says, and gives me the name of the doctor in charge. "Tell

them to call him when you go upstairs." I really assume it's the flu, but . . .

I wait for Doctor Bulkin and as soon as she appears, or almost as soon, I'm not *that* changed, I mumble about her calling "downstairs." "Oh, that," she says, "it's nothing, don't worry about it!" I'm amazed, and pleased. Later I mumble something about worrying and she cuts me off.

"It's natural," she says, "not pleasant, but normal." I know.

She tells me she suspects it's pleurisy, but she'll look at the X-rays tomorrow. Again I am overwhelmed at the care I get, even to her having gone behind a closed door and called Dr. Markham before she saw me.

So I go off, wondering whether there was some special providence that made Mark order the X-rays today, or chance, or good medicine (also, the mind being what it is, that it could have been the next week and then I wouldn't have had anything). But superstition still going strong, I leave, and at ten minutes of the hour, walk right into the Manhattan bus, which for some reason stops three blocks short of Fifty-fourth Street on the way down to leave me off at Fifty-seventh Street where I walk right onto my crosstown bus. "My luck has changed," I tell myself, "everything is okay now."

Vic is out of town, dripping with a nose cold, and I feel only faintly guilty when he calls to note that I am safely and warmly at home with only a faint pain in my chest, while he . . . Am I an invalid or am I not?

I sleep ten hours, waking only once to hold my chest when I cough. In the morning Mark grounds me for a week and I don't protest. As Jan says, "It's come to something when we're overjoyed you *only* have pneumonia, or a broken leg," but it's true. Everything is relative.

Until the next time. (And there will be one, alas, there will be one.)

·   ·

February 9. Still in purdah. I feel fine, just a little limp, but I am behaving myself. I have an idea I couldn't manage too much activity anyway, but I don't know whether I am limp from doing nothing, or limp because I *can't* do anything. Academic. Here I stand, I can do no other.

But my psyche is fraying a little. My friend Janet called to say goodbye before going on a cruise and discussed her coming varied travel plans, and we—if we are lucky—will go housekeep again with the grandchildren for a week in April. I felt very put upon. I wanted to be picked up and have my life rearranged so I can see Katmandu and Turkestan—or at least Greece and Sicily and Florence. Part of the fantasy of what one would do if one is told one has (I always get onto "one's" in this mood) X days to live. I've been thinking about the latter. Have I been told? More than anyone else? And if so, what does the world owe me because of it? Answer—nothing. It's a nasty state to get into a—a sort of the world owes me a living feeling.

It passed, of course, but I was put out with myself for recognizing it in me. Also talked to Jan last night—she was worried when Vic told her I was going to have X-rays—and I realize that in a way she thinks of it as being much worse than it is. Or at least, whenever she lets it out, which is rarely, she really has me on the other side of that line—where, at the moment, I do not feel I am.

I need to look at a picture. Or a Greek statue with an archaic smile. I am weary of contemplating my navel. Although as I write it, I note that I see the scar around it, and have no reaction whatsoever to it—I acknowledge it as mine, part of me, and perfectly ordinary.

So.

Anne Sexton: *The Awful Rowing Toward God,* "Courage"

> Later,
> when you face old age and it's a natural conclusion
> your courage will still be shown in the little ways,
> each spring will be a sword you'll sharpen,
> those you love will live in a fever of love,

and you'll bargain with the calendar
and at the last moment
when death opens the back door
you'll put on your carpet slippers
and stride out.

February 10. Back to the notebook. What brings me here to-day is the story in the *Times* about breast cancer and chemother-apy, the Italian experiment. I read it to the end, recognize one of the drugs as mine, and then see the paragraph that says chemo-therapy is being used experimentally with cancers of the ovary (first time I've seen it mentioned, usually the stories talk about uterine or cervical), colon, prostate, and bladder, cancers which have a high rate of occurrence, or re-occurrence, I should say. Or rather, *they* say. I am interested in my reaction, which is not so much blank as one of equanimity. Sure, I think, that's why the chemotherapy and it's going to work, just as, apparently, it is "working" (they do hedge so, not prevention, but no more occur-rence so far is how they put it) in the cancer of the breast tests.

My lack of fear in this is so strange, contrasted with the pan-ics I get in over so many other things, among them, waiting for a chest X-ray to be read. I am in a panic about the book—two early reviews so far, one ecstatic, one denigrating. If I could, I would buy up all the copies (I think) and burn them. The fact is that I am a different person now from when I wrote the book last spring, and I'm not sure I would —or could—do it now. Doctor Gleid-man put his finger on it in a way when he said he would like to see what I wrote *after* surgery because he was sure it would be dif-ferent. But now I'm at a new stage—a year has passed, after all—and I am not purged, at rock bottom, full of the sense that all that matters is truth, and love, and a nakedness to life. And my return to timidity is compounded by the fact that the reviews, whether laudatory or critical, don't get the point of the book *at all*. The re-viewers read it as a cliché, instead of an attempt to show that life is tragic, there are no villains—oh, well, let me not go into literary rambling here. But the truth is I wasn't sure I would live to see this one, and now I am here, and what I thought I was doing apparently isn't evident. I am also aware of how unimportant the whole thing is—not a bang, but a whimper—but it is important to me. (I'm waffling. I saw it as a tribute to Vic essentially, to his humanness and honesty and essential goodness, and instead, as I said, he emerges as cliché. And I am in the same bind now. What I am compelled to write is the story of this last year; I think it is honest, as honest, at least as I can make it, but who knows how it will come out? As sentimentality? Banal? I know, I know. I told Gottlieb I hated the rave review of which he was so proud because it didn't get the point and he said, "Oh, well, if you want a review that understands your book, you can wait throughout eternity.")

I went to a meeting last night. Women's Ink, a new, sort of feminist gathering of free-lance women writers—Betty Friedan, Eleanor Perry, Eve Merriam (all graying) and me the only ones of our age, and then perhaps a twenty-year jump to the booted, jeaned, alarming young, with only a couple of Gael Greenes and Lois Goulds to bridge the gap. There were probably about forty of us, in a large living room, smoke so heavy my eyes watered the whole time, and I have rarely felt so out of anything. At the end, though, I did walk up to Friedan and introduce myself and was pleased that she knew me and what I had written, and I did talk to a few other women. But mostly I felt as if I lived on another planet—which I do—and I wonder how much of that feeling I would have had before, and how much of it is due to my current isolation. (Waffling again—my sense of impermanence. They were talking about how to get grants, editors, agents, all the on-going minutiae of professional writing: I would have wanted only to share feelings. Like my panic at the upcoming book.)

I have been trying to "write" some of these journal episodes. Very difficult. But I have a sense—have I said this before?—I have to do it now, or not at all. Because if I stay well, on the plateau so to speak, the emotion is gone, and this is one emotion difficult to recollect in tranquility. Whereas if I don't stay well, if I have any pain, say, I won't be able to do it all. Because what I have to bear witness to now (is that "have to" a kind of hubris, maybe only a sense of what I am? I don't know) is living in a truce.

(Clinical record—for the record—having had the back, flu, and now the pleuritis, which does hang on, I find myself feeling glum and ingrown, sometimes, but not cancerous—I love that adjective, it's really murderous. It's as if reality supersedes possibility.)

My scalp is scaly—that upset me yesterday. Is it a prelude to hair loss? Well, as I have said before, I have a lot. But I hope not.

I also, for one day, had an inflammation of my Achilles heel, occasioned by getting up from a chair and standing up, honestly, just like that. But luck was with me. It happened the day before I had to see Doctor McCarthy, so he not only cut my fungoid toenail but identified the inflammation, gave me a pad to put in my shoe, and cured it! On the instant. I think his sister is not well. He kept asking me how I was, and looked sad.

I was also wiped out by last night's meeting. Slept until eight thirty without stirring. Am I weak or just unaccustomed? Could be the two glasses of wine I gulped down, too, though—I had to get liquid to wash the smoke from my throat, and there was no water around.

These entries prove my point. We are in the recitative stage of my chemotherapy journal. Boring to write about, but little spirits that haunt this place, let it be so. I have no wish to live in interesting times just so I can write about them. The price is a bit high.

Going through an old notebook I just found some notes on reactions to book number two's appearance in 1969—"the awful silence—except for Vic remembering, at three a.m., that it was the day. Capsule book review from a friend to whom I sent it—'It's fascinating, same style, but I was disappointed, I didn't laugh this time!'—hah! More on the ambivalence of people's reactions—this one was *A Loving Wife,* about the woman who has an affair— ending with 'So what is designed to communicate, *excommunicates!' Plus ça change,* etc."

More notations:

"Terminal sickness, the mark of Cain!"

Re Pascal's warning of how we waste our time "trying to be someone else." Waste our time—what a clangorous phrase, our time is all there is!

Query to Vic (in the middle of his wood): "If you knew you were going to die, what would you regret—the money you didn't make, the people you didn't help, etc.?"

Vic: "Not at all. What I didn't do—but not even that, I've had a happy life, we've done all we could do."

Query to me: "Some regret, not at what I didn't do, but at my character. I should have had a lighter heart—some are born light-hearted, some achieve it, some have it thrust upon them, let there be light-heartedness!"

And so it goes, on and on . . .

Why do I note any of it?

Because I am astonished to see that Alkeran, et al., haven't changed the essential cells. I was the same groper—about the same subjects—seven years ago as I am now. (And as illiterate in the privacy of my own pen!)

I even have pages about suicide—conclusion—"a hostile act!" Yes, Virginia, two and two indeed make four. Sometimes.

February 23, 1976. My birthday. A milestone. Two milestones. Conveniently I got out of the hospital after the first surgery on my birthday. So instead of cringing at age, I see it as a victory.

Spent it seeing Mark, and the X-ray department—as well as going to a movie and supper with Jane, Vic being in Washington.

The pleuritis seems to be the same, nonabsorbed. I am baffled. Back, chest, are these to be the little foxes? For me, who never had anything before?

I hope so.

But I still have the persistent feeling that I am being a hypochondriac, cheating somehow. Can X-rays lie? I cannot get used to the me of hospitals, doctors, medications. And when Mark asks me how I feel, I am reluctant to name symptoms. Not that I have so many, but even to admit of breathlessness, fullness in the chest, occasional pain in the back behind my ribs (I'm naming here, for the record) seems wrong. One should not complain; one should not notice; one should carry on, etc. And I keep feeling that I'm malingering when I curtail.

Actually I only just realized yesterday—after the third series of X-rays—why I'm getting them. Because I can't take the medication if there's an infection to be fought, and of course Mark has to know. It's not oversolicitude on his part.

Have to make dinner. Realized while marketing earlier that I've even cut back on cooking. I do the minimum. Period. Do I feel guilty? Not particularly.

March 1. Back from chemotherapy, and feeling better—emotionally—than I have in some weeks. How come? I'm going to try to trace what happened on that office visit to make a difference.

First, why have I been feeling flat? I don't know, truthfully. Vic asked me last night while we were driving home and I tried to find out, talking so much that finally, laughing, I simply stopped. "It's not a good idea," I told him, "because once you push the button, I simply pour out." Some of the reasons—anxiety about the book (nothing to do with this); possibly tiredness from medication (Mark last week said it was a possibility); the pleurisy which manifests itself only as a kind of heaviness in my chest, and breathlessness, but which I guess also has its debilitating effect; the incessant pounding of the word "cancer" in newspaper, magazine, TV, etc., which makes it almost impossible to escape. For example: Friday night we tuned into a "love story-comedy" in which the protagonists turned out to have leukemia and melanoma, one each; Saturday night a comedy skit in which someone was killed ended with, "Don't worry, she found out she had cancer"; *Nova* introduced the story of the double helix with its relationship to cancer research; and so on, ad infinitum. Added to what goes on in my head (which I am trying to "write out," to get rid of it, in a sense), no wonder I get tired. But then as we were driving, a sentence came up from nowhere, the way it may in a psychiatrist's room: "I'm scared because I'm not getting my shots."

I told Mark the latter—how I was lonely for Fluorouracil, for God's sake—and he understood that it's not so much the medication as the upset routine that bothers me. And that's true. I seem to have worked out a pattern that I have adjusted to, and so long as I don't have to think about it, simply follow the pattern, I'm okay. Any deviation—and this is not only true medically—requires a new adaptation. So he gave me my two shots—maybe he would have anyway, I don't know—and I was relieved. It's a very delicate balance—when not to order tests, when to take something seriously, when to overlook, I'm not sure it can be figured out, it has to be intuited.

And then we talked, and I found our talk very exciting and reassuring. For my own reasons obviously, I cling to the notion that no one really knows anything for sure, and that statistics don't apply to individuals. Mark said that it used to be that only condemned criminals knew for a certainty the date of their deaths (even that, I realize now, wasn't 100 percent, there could always, à la Brecht, be a last-minute pardon, or an earthquake, or something), but that now science can fairly estimate the progress of an illness. But then he went on to cite example after example within his own experience where it didn't turn out to be so—the woman with cancer of the pancreas who was alive three years after her six-month span was up; the woman with "a few weeks" to live and many metastases who was back at work in a month or two, and so on and so. He told of cancer tumors that remain in status quo even when they are too big for surgery; of juvenile tumors that actually change character; of research that shows that changes in DNA, once thought irreversible, may actually be reversed; of experiments with plants and fish that give great promise.

It wasn't the detail, it was his sharing of his own hope and optimism that made me understand for the first time how he can work in oncology without being overwhelmed. Sure, people die of cancer, but other people don't, or live much longer than one would expect. And he told me how he expects changes in treatment to come about soon—okay, maybe not in my lifetime (or his), but the feeling in that small examining room was that it would be *soon* (for us), and it's the feeling that's so important, the feeling that has always been there, which is not composed of fudging or lying (he even said, "You know all the treatments we have now have destructive elements—surgery, radiation, chemotherapy"), but an honesty that takes in the positive as well as the negative. (Why do we always ascribe to truth-telling the faculty of doling out unpleasant facts? "I love you" is as true as "I hate you"; sometimes, even more true.)

We also talked again a little about death and dying—a repeat conversation, sure, but some things have to be said over and over again, I find, because the context always changes. And again I saw that "dying" is as uncertain a word as anything else ("death" I understand, and that doesn't scare me, never has, I don't think ever will. I perceive it as "nonbeing"—I just looked at what I wrote—"Death I understand"—I mean just the opposite, death I don't understand, and don't expect to, and it really doesn't concern me, I work at my own immortality—which is to be understood, I guess—in the here and now)—the last "quotation mark," as Mark has said—as long as you're alive, you're not dying, I guess, or are dying, which may amount to the same thing.

So how much does "intervention" affect a patient? A physician's attitude? Well, I'm not in crisis, waiting for radiation (just a dopy Friday X-ray which has nothing to do with anything), or anything else—as a matter of fact, listening to Mark's stories of women who come to the hospital in extremis and leave to go home and resume their duties, I feel, as usual, somewhat malingering even to give the matter any thought—BUT—it is my opinion that attitudes (i.e., loving kindness) do more than medication can to justify God's ways to man.

End of garbled report (in my next life I shall take at least one course in chemistry and biology so that I can understand what I am told, or at least find the words to translate my understanding —I got away with geology and physics! None of which apply—I think).

March 2. Living on three levels—reality, the journal, and a not-too-successful attempt to make quasi-fiction of the fact recorded here. This morning, I think, the three intersected. I awoke with a start, frightened by a dream in which I was looking into the toilet and saw a rim of blood around my stool. First dream of symptoms ever.

Explanation is simple though. I have been trying to write about the *idée fixe,* so it's been in my mind more. Sometime last week the *Times* had a story out of Rome about vitamin C interfering with the accuracy of a test physicians use to find blood in stools before it is actually visible to the eye. (Why did I notice it? Because all such stories appear printed in capital letters, of course, and because I didn't know blood had a *non*-visible state.) I wasn't at all conscious of having been upset by it or even remembering it. But . . . And—in all reality—I am aware of my body in a rather undercutting way. I feel heavy, literally; haven't gotten used to the extra poundage I lug around. My chest seems about the same—just enough to make me puff occasionally, mild discomfort when I sneeze, say. Enough already. And since I am inactive because of the foregoing, my stomach sags and my back twinges. All of it unimportant, all of it profoundly to be settled for. But I keep having this image—or at least I do now, as I write—of the lithe, ache-free, *running* person I used to be (was I?), and I want to call out, "Come back! I'm here!" Am I? Will she? A few more weeks, I think, and it will be all right. It seems to me that the last two years have been a history of just about getting there, and then getting tripped by back, surgery, flu, whatever. I feel like a child learning to walk, up on my feet, then flop, then try again. And how did I get off on this tack? I don't know. I know. It's foggy and rainy out. Pathetic fallacy. Always happens. It smacks of self-pity, when I know, gratefully and apprehensively, that I couldn't be luckier for that to have been all. (Business of placating evil eye—please, kid, I'll settle for it, don't think I'm complaining.)

March 8. So it begins again. Tests. And the superstitions pour in—also as usual.

On the way for my shots I remembered I had forgotten to bring this month's journal. First time. And I had thought that I had been right in assuming about a month ago—after a year of it —that we were at a new stage, and that I should start trying to write it for one of two reasons—it will go on as it is, so new insights will be fewer, or it will not, and I will be unable to write.

Which it will be I still don't know. I hurt sitting here—as I did last June with my back, although not quite as much—and so I don't know how much of the fear and—what is the word? disillusion, almost—I feel is due to that. Anyway I'm in the same trap— I really think I'm all right (but why does the fluid stay in my chest? I'm not so worried about the back because it comes and goes, and I've been through it all year, on and off).

So I note ironies (or superstitions):

—The one X-ray I wasn't "afraid of" was the chest one. What could be the matter with my chest! (Somewhere in recent weeks I saw a cancer patient described in which "fluid in the chest" was mentioned, but I passed over it in my mind. I still don't know what it could mean.)

—Yesterday I bought "advance" groceries in the Arab store on Atlantic Avenue—and had the fleeting feeling of tempting fate, i.e., would I use up two pounds of pilaff?

—We had our "last" weekend—Kathy, Hilary, Vic, and I. It was supposed to be Kathy's, pre-baby, and we did all kinds of things we wouldn't have otherwise. Whose "last" was it really?

—I bought some spring clothes—as yet unworn—larger size.

—The Sarasota apartment is probably rented till next year, someone looked at the house yesterday and expressed interest, first such interest since it's been on sale. I feel being closed in upon.

—My brother's call saying he wants to come to see me during his spring vacation. He was uneasy about me. I wrote that I'd like to see him but not because I'm sick, because I'm well.

—My sister is coming east to stay a week April 15.

—And, of course, we spent much time over the weekend discussing how I could help Kathy with the baby. End of May. I told Mark I hoped I would be well enough by then—meaning end of back (which in a way has been plaguing me on and off since New Year's). So he linked these tests he's ordering to "having them over with by May." So—liver, bone, IVP, I presume GI and barium enema (if I'm lucky, if the other tests don't show anything!).

Am I scared? Sure. But this time, more discouraged than scared. I hate the hospital setting. It used to be interesting, no more. I hate the time it takes. I hate not being able to forget about the whole thing and go on with living.

Interesting note: The book should have arrived last week. I am so uninterested I haven't even called to find out what's the matter. Obviously it can't come out as scheduled, it's so far behind, but it seems very unimportant. Natural? I don't know. Jacqueline Susann went on tours pushing hers while she was dying, of breast cancer apparently—so did Connie Ryan with his.

Do I think anything will be found? I know enough by now to know I just don't know. Just get through the limbo. Tests this week, I hope the rest (if there is a rest, and I hope so, I guess) early next week, and may I then be able again to try to go and sin no more . . . It still *is* strange that I felt I had better get started writing it before it was too late. I have three stories done. All the rest to do . . . Isn't it strange how I try to make patterns where clearly there can be none? Am I scaring myself with stories about wolves to make sure they really don't come true?

.   .

March 11.

> And set me down
> Today. Tonight. Through my
> Invisible new veil
> Of finity, I see
> November's world—
> Low scud, slick street, three giggling girls—
> As, oddly, not as sombre
> As December,
> But as green
> As anything:
> As spring.—Sissman

I lost a friend today—L. E. Sissman. He was forty-eight, and he had fought the Hodgkin's since 1965. As always, I am surprised that people die—somehow I think that if they think right (as he did) and have super care (as he must have), they make it. But in his last essay, I think, he sounded tired. Maybe it was time. Anyway, even though it was only a few letters, I was looking forward to sending him the book, as he had asked, and eventually (daydream) talking to him. Sic transit. (Alas, wryly, there goes my own chance of getting a *New Yorker* review, too.) I feel guilty reading the obit. He not only wrote his poems and articles, he still worked in an advertising agency when he died. I wrote his wife, thanking her for making him possible. (I don't think we can do it alone.) My fantasies of it being easier if I didn't have to think about bothering Vic—worry, that is—evaporate as soon as something goes wrong. It was so nice to have my back rubbed when it went into spasm, so special to be driven up yesterday. I hope Mark was right—that there is a joy in the giving. But even though I don't think I keep Vic from doing anything—I try not to—it must be a drag, a fearful drag, sitting through the tests, watching the back. I'm sorry.

I don't know how I got started on the foregoing. I guess because I hate in any way being the "invalid" wife. I try not to be, don't really perceive myself as such, but am I?

Tests on. For some reason, I am not as afraid or pushed as I was last writing. The hospital has its own momentum, and everyone is very nice. The technician this time gave me times when phases would be over, told me I could move my head when that part was done. Small bits, but a far cry from the first time, when I felt abandoned in the dark.

And, of course, for the record, Doctor Bulkin couldn't have been kinder. Naturally when I saw Doctor Haberman, the spasm that had me immobilized and in pain for forty minutes the night before was practically nonexistent. In the morning I couldn't bend to brush my teeth; in his office, I could get within six inches of my toes. Typical. But he still ordered massive doses of Valium and aspirin which *do* leave me practically symptom-free—so I'll juggle them.

Is my calmness Valium? Alas, could be.

I still keep feeling like a hypochondriac. As though *I* am ordering the tests, and on false pretenses. I have to tell myself that I did (do?) have cancer, that I am on chemotherapy, that last time the tests showed something (but it turned out somewhat all right), that obviously I have to be checked, and that furthermore there is a symptom—the fluid in my chest. It just struck me that it could have been there *before,* the flu, and not connected. Oh, well. The usual mental processes. If it's something, it's early.

But I don't feel as if it's anything.

Please let Kathy have her baby without any hassle from me.

March 17. I was "lucky." IVP, liver and bone scans normal, so Mark ordered the barium and GI series. (Wonder what he can think of next?) As usual, I hate to go to Montefiore, hate waiting around and then find such skill and kindness I don't ever want to go anywhere else. This time it was my old friend Rodriguez who took my sheet from somewhere else and did the IVP for me.

(Story: He did the last chest X-ray, at which time there was a one-hundred-and-two-year-old woman ahead of me screaming and yelling. Turned out she was senile, of course, but doughty, and when he touched her pelvic area she practically accused him of rape and said her "husband wouldn't like it." He had been horrified but I thought it was marvelous. Conversation continued during the IVP —or at least before—turns out he's been divorced, is good friends with ex-wife and her new husband, and is baffled by changes in Puerto Rican culture in re sex. Bad sentence, interesting conversation.)

Read Book of Esther over weekend prior to telling the kids the story (for the record, a self-serving bitch, decided not to tell kids about her), and then stumbled onto Book of Job. Will not insult even myself by including commentary on Book of Job except to state that the last two years have notably increased my understanding of same. I even love the preposterous ending. No one can live on the plane that precedes it on any sustained level. You have to have a bit of fairy story—or hope. (Noted in Montefiore elevator a sign in Spanish that seems to indicate that "wait" and "hope" have the same root. Asked Rodriguez about it, and it's so.)

As a footnote to the Book of Job: I notice since the tests began I use Saran Wrap. Very significant. I am exceedingly chintzy about Saran Wrap, belonging to a waxpaper generation. But a carpe diem quality has taken over.

I am glad about the barium enema (Dr. Ben told me it was okay). Also told me he saw two little clips inside me. "From the first surgery or the second?" "Second." I told Vic and he said he knew about it. They're a marker apparently. Good sign. If there's nothing suspicious between them, it means status quo. I hope. The upper area, obviously, is the one where I had trouble (or didn't, although it showed). But I am glad to be spared tubes and bags, which I assume are the pitfalls of the lower bowel area.

Thursday to go.

I was upset last night because Mildred called from Washington in her usual panic to find out "what's the matter" and "how the tests are going." It seems Vic told Richard on Sunday when he spoke to him, and he told Mildred. (I was also upset that Vic had told Richard, then realized he must be upset and of course should be able to talk to a friend. He is not sleeping well either, and I guess he's worried, which makes me feel very guilty. I try not to be a holding-down wife—encourage him to play poker, for instance—and I don't think I keep him from doing anything, or us from doing anything, but how do I know? I don't.) I didn't realize she knew at first and kept saying I was fine so she kept pushing. I had tried not to tell anyone, although Vic did tell Jan when she was in the office, and she told Kathy, but so far as they know, the barium one was it. What bothered me about Mildred's call was that I told her all the tests were negative and I was fine, and since there are more to go, I felt I was tempting fate. (Sorry. But this has to be a record.)

Back pretty much okay except for a minor setback last night. We went to make a condolence call on an elderly friend (husband died at ninety) and she came to sit beside me, started to fall toward my left, sacroiliacal side, I grabbed her—and wrenched the muscle again. But Valium and aspirin and a night's rest apparently fixed it.

Just read a review of *Kinflicks*. Part of the plot apparently concerns a dying mother's reassessment of her life, philosophy, etc., during her lengthy dying. I know I'm not dying (okay, let's not go into the semantics of that), but it seems to me that really one (here we go, when it becomes touchy, "I" become "one") is more involved with Saran Wrap than reassessments of one's philosophy. I should not have thought so as an observer, but that's how it seems when you're in it.

Or maybe I'm not in it. I'll let you know.

March 23. Still in limbo—somewhat. Tests as of Friday all okay—Vic reported Mark had said it was "the best news yet," but to me, truthfully, Mark said he didn't know why the chest remains in status quo. Disliking myself, I found myself pushing Mark to the wall—i.e., "But you don't think it's anything, do you?"—and he, of course, said he didn't know. If he did, I wouldn't be seeing a chest man Thursday. I'm glad he doesn't respond to pressure for fake reassurances because I wouldn't believe them anyway. Why do I do it? (I keep thinking about the chest—I don't see how it can be anything much—it started so acutely and then got better and I don't feel anything now. Still.)

Generally, of course, I'm relieved. Mark also said to Vic that he thought I was under "great emotional pressure," although I didn't show it. Well, the pressure came and went. Worse away from the hospital somehow than in it—maybe because everyone is so kind and matter of fact, and I am so much better off than the people around me waiting for X-rays. I wonder if Plato was right in his theory that his ideal state would have to have doctors who themselves had suffered the diseases they treated. Well, just stating it makes the answer obvious—it's ridiculous. But a little footnote about Dr. Ben WHO LETS YOU KNOW AS HE GOES ALONG. Somehow in all the chit-chat I mentioned my Purim story of Esther and then that I had read Job. Said he, "The last time I read it was a couple of years ago when I was going through a very bad time." Amid all the jokes.

This is going to be disjointed for two reasons—I'm still waiting for Thursday, and I should have written it day by day. So just some notes:

—I keep wondering if I would be as anxious (sure I was anxious) if I had only myself to think about. Not that I'm unselfish. On the contrary. My self-absorption is frightening. (A few minutes ago I called someone to leave a message about a meeting I couldn't get to, and when she refused to take the message but told me to call the secretary and gave me the number, I thought afterward that she would have taken it if she "had known." My God.) I worry about being repulsive, sickly, burdensome, etc. Was relieved when the barium enema was okay (I think—more of that later), because *that* surgery wouldn't be necessary. Find myself thinking the lungs are, at least, tidy and inner.

But then I realize, or at least think, that if I were alone, I wouldn't be here in the first place. If there is some inner fight going on, and I think there is, I wouldn't be fighting. I still think I didn't fight a few years ago, and so got started. (None of this presumes to be scientific or sensible—I'm just trying to pry out what goes on in my mind at this time, unprettied up.)

When I say to Vic I am sorry I'm putting him through this, he looks at me in astonishment. "Wasn't I in bed for three months last summer?" True, but that was different. It was going to end. He points out I go about my business, even to cooking his dinners. True. But that's not what impresses me. It's one sentence—"But I want to take care of you." It truly seems to come from the heart. And on Sunday I read a review of an autobiography by Helen Bevington in which she tells of her husband living five years with cancer and says, "I knew he was going to die, but I am grateful to him for living that long."

—I mull over why all philosophy goes by the board during the weeks of tests. Well, not all. Some of the days I really wasn't worried at all, and, looking back, I think it's when my back hurt and I took Valium at night. Which is the real me, with Valium or without? As a matter of principle, I didn't take it unless I had to —and not at all with the castor oil, milk of magnesia tests. By Thursday when I couldn't have any because of the barium for the EI tests, I was calm. Cynically so, in a way (I fight, I think, because I feel I have to be hopeful to help myself). I thought what difference does it make (which is always true, of course), and that it might be better to get it all over with instead of engaging in this endless holding battle, and that I am, when I think about it, as dispensable as anyone I can think of. I have very few loose ends, barring a few stories I could finish, and how important are they? Jan and Kathy and their families will have perfectly good lives with or without me, they're doing fine, I am of no use to them except just to be. In terms of them I have achieved *sannyasi*—the

Hindu state in which you are to go into the woods after you have seen your grandchildren and start loosening yourself from life. As far as Vic is concerned, he can—and I think will—have another life, a second life, younger and gayer. And so it goes—having written the foregoing I find myself a little tearful, and shocked, I *thought* it, but getting it down, I see it's true, I am really not essential to anyone and, potentially, only a burden. (I HATE the foregoing, but that's what I thought, may still think . . .) Okay, what goes on? Nothing new, I see. I don't know what I'm hiding, but on the surface, I'm the same as I always was, seeing myself only reflected back from other people. The question is, I guess, am I of use to myself? Is my life worth living to *me?* As much as ever? The answer comes out "more so," but I don't know if that's phony. I think I can only respond in the here and now to that—I can't think of a time when life was essentially better, in terms of inner questions, that is, there were always doubts. Now I can write, "I want to take care of you," and know it's so—back to the old merry-go-round, responding in terms of someone else—how about *me?* If only I behaved better—*thought* better, that is—I'd settle for me right now. With only a spot of vanishing pleurisy, please . . .

—Re how much I "know" about my physical status, and how much I don't. I was surprised when Dr. Ben said the barium enema results were "better." I don't think I knew that it had been questionable last time, but I must have. Why else the proctoscope? I think I must hear what I want to hear. No, I don't think that's the process. I think what I do is ask a question, listen to part of the answer, and then interrupt with the rest of the "answer" myself, with the result that I never really get a complete answer. My doing. Whether it is intentional or not, I'm not sure. I think what I do is shy away from words—"metastasis," for instance. I think of cells floating around, which are being (have been?) licked.

I did have a turn watching a bit of the GI films when I was on my right side. A black mass kept swirling like pictures of the growth of cancer cells that I saw on *Nova* a couple of weeks ago.

Dr. Ben explained it was the barium going through that I was seeing. (I didn't tell him what it had looked like to me.) If you want
to know how I feel about cancer cells, I shall tell you. I don't feel
invaded. Maybe I would if I had a growing mass, but as it is, I
feel rather friendly toward such of them as there are. I think of
them as damaged, inferior creatures that don't want to be there any
more than I want them, and that somehow, with the shots and the
pills and my own good cells, we are transforming them into fine
upright healthy kids. I feel protective toward them, as if they were
outside of the real me, not part of me.

   —Last time a series was finished and okay (What am I saying? The last series wasn't okay at all. What the devil *is* the
mind?)—anyway, the times the tests *were* okay, I felt released.
Radiant. Now—with Thursday in mind perhaps—I feel pleased,
relieved but resigned. One day at a time. I do begin to have the
feeling I am going to get away with it—go on and on—but it
will, nevertheless, always be a presence. Enhancing in some ways,
as I have noted before and still feel—but a pain in the ass too,
thank you.

   Please—only pleurisy on Thursday!

   Footnote to above: Just got a telephone call from Vic. Do I
mind going to Florida on Christmas Day next year—it falls on a
Saturday? I listen to him bemused. "No," I say, "not at all."
"Okay," he says. "Do you want to take the nine o'clock plane or
the ten o'clock plane?" "Ten o'clock," I say. "But don't you have
reservations for Puerto Rico?" I had learned this from Jan. "Yes,"
he says. "In case."

   March 26. Well, it's not just a "little pleurisy." Maybe. As I
had expected really, Dr. Blumberg, the chest doctor, did not wave
a wand and say forget it, it's nothing. He did not really seem to
take it too seriously, except to say it could be any one of ten manifestations ranging from a clot (I did have a little something in
my right leg, come to think of it), tuberculosis (because I am

"vulnerable" to infection, he doesn't know about my bloods, I guess), medication, edema, heart, tumor, etc. Of course I asked him about "tumor." "It's not my first guess," he said. Two-sided, apparently. Oh, yes, also, pleurisy. Maybe I didn't have flu, but pleurisy. (Memo to Mark—okay, okay, next time you suggest my seeing a "doctor" when I have something, I will.) Heart, I thought of. That's okay. Symptoms? Negligible—rarely, mostly in bed in the morning or late at night, five or six times maybe in a year that I can recall, there is this thin long burning worm of pain (which usually ends up seeming to be associated with gas). He did ask my family history, and I don't know whether I had suppressed this earlier, but I was surprised to have to recall that the only brothers of my father I ever knew both died of cancer, one in his fifties, one in his late seventies. Also that a cousin I don't know has had a malignancy, uterine. I seem to trace my family history only to my mother's side because I knew them so well. What else did I pick up? He watched me come into his office and commented that I "ran"; asked me how I got there (to see how much walking I did), and remarked that he was reluctant to interfere with "success." From which I gather he thought I was doing well—even so.

Which I suppose I am. I have been rather sour the last few days, and almost cynical since I saw Dr. Blumberg. I imagine I will either have more probes, surely more X-rays, and the least that will happen is "I will be watched." So all it amounts to is that next to the big sword hanging over my head is perhaps a small dagger. What's the difference? I also tell myself that to be sour in any way is to be most ungrateful, since compared to other patients I am in clover itself. And maybe there's the rub. "Patients." I don't like to think of myself as a "patient," and don't, until my nose is rubbed in it.

I have talked to Vic about all of this more than I have in the past. It doesn't seem to throw him. He has his own timetable. "Five years of watching before you can be called cured." Hah! Walking through a liquor store nearby last night, just browsing, he got into conversation with the salesman, who pointed to some bottles that would be good to buy now for use five years hence. "How about it?" asked Vic. "That's up to you," I said. "If you think you'll need them. What I'm interested in is a bottle I can drink today." "I just wanted to know your state of mind," replied Vic. Farewell to Pollyanna.

You want to know something? Just writing the foregoing paragraph made me grin. As if a load had rolled off my shoulders somehow. It's a comfort sometimes not to be sweetness and light.

March 29. Peace. For now.

I was not only tense and depressed all weekend but I ached in my chest. I acknowledged the same rather wryly, for if in my private bargaining I swap cancer for heart, the understanding is that it shall be painless and noninterfering. Also had bad dreams. Alas, I forget all but one—I broke a vial of Fluorouracil I needed! Kept waking up at five thirty every morning. Got more and more ingrown.

Saw Mark on Monday. No chest pains. (Also, my thin hot little worm is not descriptive of angina, he informed me—which makes sense, because *that* I have had on rare occasion for many, many years. Gas. Or tension.) Less (as I write this, I become aware of it) back pain. Why? Not so much what he says, but what I pick up. No particular sweat. This time. After two (!) years, I am again reassured and reinforced by realization of his attitude toward treatment, tests, etc. We are not, at this time, to have chest punctures or biopsies (very important matter, the last—he lets drop he doesn't think anything would be found) because there is no reason to do a test unless one is going to do something about it. He also mentions a seventy-five-year-old patient with terminal emphysema and his (Mark's) unhappiness at the tubing and indignities the man may be subjected to, in the name of what? (As I listen, I apply it to myself. We do, you know, friend M. And I am glad. A load goes. Again, it's not death, it's the process to which one is forced to submit. Mark wouldn't have it done to me. Good.) Also,

I can go to Florida. And take my medication with me. So nothing is changed, physically, but in my head, everything is.

(The above reminded me that I had just read in *The American Scholar* a quotation from Pliny: "I do not indeed hold that life ought to be so prized that by any and every means it should be prolonged. You holding this view, whoever you are, will nonetheless die . . . Of all the blessings given to man by nature none is greater than a timely death."

Also, from Freud: "Much is won if we succeed in transforming hysterical misery into common unhappiness," i.e., not Utopia, just day-to-day life is what we settle for.

Also, engraved on William Hazlitt's gravestone: "Contented and Grateful."

Thank you, *American Scholar*. Nice pickings for ten minutes of browsing.)

I have been thinking about an article in the *Times* today about Orville Kelly, cancer patient, founder of Make Today Count (story lead: "A cancer patient who may be dying of his disease"— was diagnosed three years ago, in recent months signs of disease have disappeared under chemotherapy). The organization has fifty-four chapters, and talking to members Kelly reports that "life is often hardly worth living for the many patients and their families who are unable to cope with the emotional and social consequences" while their lives are prolonged by modern cancer treatments. "The fear, depression, sexual problems and anger were often more difficult to contend with than the cancer itself," Kelly says.

Suddenly I feel like the Molière character who discovers he has been talking prose all his life. Ah, so. I have apparently been taking for granted my freedom from what Kelly says cancer victims complain of (in 25,000 letters to him alone)—"deception," "dishonest relatives who refuse to admit they have cancer," lack of communication, rejection by friends, etc.

Item: No one has deceived me (except perhaps on occasion, I, myself).

Item: There is nothing I cannot say to Vic, to Jan, to Kathy, my sons-in-law, my relatives, my real friends—*if* I so chose. If I censor, it is not to trouble them, but even then, they make it clear they are less troubled if I am as honest with them as I can be.

Item: Except for the brief period after the hysterectomy, I never have felt physically rejected by Vic, and that was a reaction to the surgery mostly, I think, and normal. On the contrary, he even makes my weight gain appear as a plus. Our circle is more constricted than it ever was, but I think there are many reasons for this, least of which is my illness. I have been less available at times (hospital, Florida, tests, etc.), but if *I* reach out, there is a response. Maybe there are others, but I can think of only one couple who perhaps are "afraid" of me, and even there, the reason may just as well lie elsewhere.

Item: My medical care (*vide* preceding pages) has always more than included my emotional state.

Item: Anger? At me? I don't feel any. (Truthfully, what I get from Jan and Kathy is admiration—"You're doing so beautifully," said Jan only yesterday—Kathy even wrote it.) From Vic? I *feel* like a burden sometimes, but I cannot honestly pick up the slightest indication from him that he feels me so (and I would, I would, that I know). Anger *from* me? At myself, for not being more heroic, yes. At the situation? I'm sure, however disguised. At anyone else? No. (Except when I felt pushed by my father that time. Or when demands that make me feel guilty are made upon me.)

I guess what I'm driving at is that this isn't *my* journal, it's *ours*. Or theirs. Looking back over the last two years, I cannot think of one instance in which Vic, Jan, or Kathy behaved in any way other than I would wish (or consider helpful to me) in relation to my—what? Condition? Illness? Whatever.

The reason I spell all this out—the reason for all the "prose" —is that I realize that what I have taken for granted as the climate in which I live is not necessarily the climate other people have. And when I change it in my mind, try to think what it would be

with deception, lack of love, a need to dissemble, rejection, etc.—
I can't think. The image I get is of me locked in a cage in the dark.

April 11. An interesting time. (The Chinese curse, of course,
to live in interesting times, but I don't know. Not entirely.)

I guess it started about ten days ago, soon after seeing Dr.
Blumberg when, naturally, I had no symptoms. I began to feel
more and more breathless and less able to walk, more and more
convinced it was something in my head. Anxious about going to
Sarasota and packing up the apartment with the little kids around;
anxious about my sister and her family coming to stay next week,
who knows? On the way to Mark's on Monday, I barely made it to
the bus, so breathless and a pain like a knife. Unfortunately by the
time I got there, I felt much better, and talking to him, alas, even
better. And when he found nothing on examination I was convinced it was all in my head. But it came and went, a block was
hard to navigate, and Wednesday night, before we were to leave
for Sarasota, kids already sleeping over, ready to leave for the airport at eight a.m., I could not breathe, had sweats, diarrhea, and
fear—I would go to Sarasota and end up in a hospital with Vic
having the kids, and Mark a thousand miles away! I finally told
Vic how I felt, after getting up for the umpteenth time, and he insisted that I had to call Mark in the morning and cancel if necessary. So, with a half hour to go, I did call (terrible thing to do, call
a doctor at 7:30 a.m., I know it), and wisely, Mark said he couldn't
tell, I had better have an X-ray. So Vic took off with my assurance
I'd be down the next day, and the new tests began. I was both startled and relieved to learn there was fluid in my chest—relieved
because it wasn't in my head and because I didn't have to go on trying to pretend everything was normal and because I hadn't gone
south where I couldn't have coped. Dr. Blumberg, like everyone,
was kind and skilled, and commented that the fluid was "nice and
clear," which I translated as a poor omen, i.e., no bacteria, no clots,
Q.E.D., cancer cells. There had been an article in the *Times* about

lung cancer that day, naturally, and I had read that it is generally inoperable in a third of the cases by the time it was found, that it was the most lethal form, that it spread to spine and brain (double-take—the backache? But that has been continuing, on and off, same place, for two years, acutely on and off, for a year, and Dr. Haberman and scans found nothing—therefore, probably not connected), and took three to six months. On the other hand, I figured, what they are talking about are tumors they can spot, and obviously nothing has been spotted with me. All of this, with, I think, genuine calm. When I am waiting for reports of tests, I'm not calm; now that there is obviously something, I am. Why? Shock? I don't think so. Waiting for the shoe to drop syndrome? Partly. Because there is nothing I can do about it? Maybe.

I also felt much much better with the fluid out. Went home by bus—no sweat. Was going to take a taxi from the bus, but took another bus instead. Broke down only to the extent of ordering milk and stuff from Gristede's inasmuch as I had emptied the refrigerator. Also, have stopped eating standing up at a kitchen counter. I put my food on a tray and eat either at a table or in the study. (The Saran Wrap syndrome.)

I slept very well.

Also came to some conclusions. Still very calm. (Have I leaped to the resignation phase? Past hope, fear, anger, etc.? Seems very premature but that may still be the mechanism.) Possibilities:

1. Since everything else is excluded (and was the next day with the heart test), it has to be cancer-related. Stray cells? Would they produce so much fluid? Is the chemotherapy no longer effective? Is this a repetition—something starts, I reject it, the fluid part of the starting process. Obviously I don't know, but I decide—

2. I will probably ("we," is more accurate) fight this off. Why not? If it's so small it's not yet visible . . . Anyway this isn't the end, probably, there are lots of avenues to go first.

3. However, if it is going to go its relentless way, I'd rather have it in the lung (although I don't like the choking feeling) than where I'd need resections and bags, etc. Also, that apparently

goes faster, and I'd rather have something fast than slow, to spare everyone.

4. I don't want to hang around indefinitely as an invalid wife. If it's fast, Vic has a chance at a new life. That doesn't upset me any more. I wish it for him.

I meet Mark in the corridor after the lung tests, he asks me how I feel, and right away I dump on him. "It's lung cancer, isn't it?" I say cheerily. I honestly don't remember what he answered, except he didn't deny it. He said he would treat me empirically—act "as if" it were, change my medication slightly. No radiation, no surgery.

So we are essentially status quo, it seems to me, except that instead of being treated generally, I have a specific medication. I remember that when all the tests were over, and negative, except for the pleural fluid, Mark said, "I wish I could tell you everything was all right, but . . ." and that, of course, is the way it has been all along. (I note I am acting as if it were a certainty but I realize it isn't 100 percent. All the tests aren't reported, it could be something else, but I doubt it.) The only question I have physically, therefore (I seem to be assuming we'll lick these cells too), is how can we keep the fluid from returning and incapacitating me? Or, knowing it's there, do you just function around it? So far, I've had no cancer symptoms to cope with; I don't know how it's going to be with this added on. Harder. Obviously.

Now, periphery—

Vic was very upset. Shocked, I think, that there was something. He kept saying, "I've never seen you like this before. You're so tense. So nervous about going." I think he was genuinely surprised to find out there was a physical basis. His first reaction was to say he would come home. I insisted that he not, for many reasons. He has to close the apartment, he needs a vacation—he'll enjoy it with the kids—and he needs the space from me, as do I from him. It is easier for me to be alone these few days, pulling myself together without having to maintain a façade.

Not that I've been very alone. I am both touched and uneasy

by the response to me. At first I wasn't going to tell anyone. Then I thought I'd better tell my sister-in-law Mollie at least that I was alone in the city. Then I told Jan, realizing I couldn't spare her knowing that I wasn't with Vic and the kids. And I called Kathy because I know she would be furious if I kept anything from her. So Jan has been over—Friday night, and just now for an hour; my friend Helen came in from the country to spend Saturday; my sister-in-law Mollie got tickets for the Liv Ullmann movie so I wouldn't have to wait in line; and a few people just called "because I've been thinking of you and got a little worried."!! And, of course, Vic calls two or three times a day. I'm uneasy because I keep thinking, what do they know I don't? Nothing, I know that —not as much. But even so . . .

I did make a mistake with Jan Friday night. I thought aloud. She is doing publicity for the American Cancer Society media awards so I know she reads what I read in the press at least, and I knew she had read the lung cancer story. So I casually said I'd prefer it to be that to bowel surgery, that I wouldn't want to hang around sick very long to be a burden, etc., that I wasn't scared particularly, that it was essentially more of the same—uncertainty, day to day, with me essentially hopeful as to prognosis, but not knowing. It scared her. She told Kathy that I was going to refuse surgery. Where she got that I have no idea, since the subject never came up, and she also apparently suggested to Kathy that she come to see me next week. What Jan told me was that Kathy had said she might come down, and I became very upset about it. My sister and family are going to be here, there's no room, I don't want Kathy traveling now, and why all the fuss? I finally brought it up with Kathy, and Kathy said it had been Jan's idea, that she was confused by the suggestion, and really didn't think it was necessary either. But then she said I had frightened Jan by the no-surgery statement. I told her I was sure I hadn't said it, but that it was true I had erred in saying that if anything happened, I'd just as soon it be quick. Said Kathy: "But I don't want you to feel that way. I want you as long as possible under any circumstances."

Much ado.

Are we making an enormous mountain of a mole hill? I have no idea.

Something inside me feels qualitatively different, but I can't tell if it's the fluid that was already there (or is more building up?), the diuretic pills, the Valium and Bufferin I just took, the lung tap, no idea. I certainly am in no panic, but I do feel in limbo. Waiting, for what I don't know. On the bus coming down Friday I made some notes: "Life as if—hope is frightening—easier without in a way—still have to fight—reality is sobering—feel 'all passion spent'—no longer, if, or when, but how—all I want is not to make it hard for anyone—hope for it not to hurt so much I can't function—I want dignity, serenity, reasonable comfort, ability to be pleasant to everyone—don't understand—but then—if we knew and understood, there would be nothing to keep us living, would there?"

Two dreams last night:

1. Wish fulfillment—someone draws last of fluid from my chest and says, "That's all it was. You're over it. Everything is the way it was before."

2. Change of status—I give Mark the pages from my journal and he gives them back to me. "I don't want them any more," he says. "You're not a patient now."

Wouldn't it be nice if it turned out to be a virus?

Postscript

Violet Weingarten stopped writing at the end of April 1976 after a lengthy and difficult hospitalization. She died at Montefiore Hospital on July 17. We were at her side. She remained alert and conscious until a few hours before her death and although uncomfortable and often frightened, she never relinquished that strength and grace that she had maintained throughout her illness. She remained involved with life, speaking of such diverse matters as the ongoing Democratic Convention and her six-week-old grandson. She was continually attempting to reassure us. She never acknowledged the extent of her illness or even indicated that she knew she was dying. Then, at the end, she said, "Forgive me, but this is absurd." She then lost consciousness and, a few hours later, died.

Reading this journal after her death was very painful for us. We discovered the extent to which she privately acknowledged the gravity of her illness. We wished we could talk with her about the opinions, insights, discoveries, fears, and humor we discovered in the journal. We missed her even more and this intensified our grief.

The decision to publish the journal was difficult. To allow the death of our wife and mother, for us a very private event, to become public was disturbing. But Violet was a writer as well as our wife and mother and we believe that she intended this journal to be published someday. And because she was a good writer, her journal should make her own experience significant to a great many people.

Victor Weingarten
Jan Greenberg
Kathy Weingarten

A Note on the Type

The text of this book was set on the Linotype in Garamond, a modern rendering of the type first cut by Claude Garamond (1510–1561). Garamond was a pupil of Geoffroy Tory and is believed to have based his letters on the Venetian models, although he introduced a number of important differences, and it is to him we owe the letter which we know as old-style. He gave to his letters a certain elegance and a feeling of movement that won for their creator an immediate reputation and the patronage of Francis I of France.

COMPOSED BY THE BOOK PRESS, BRATTLEBORO, VERMONT
PRINTED AND BOUND BY THE HADDON CRAFTSMEN,
SCRANTON, PENNSYLVANIA
DESIGNED BY GWEN TOWNSEND